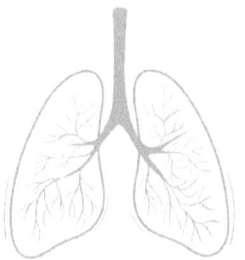

ISBNs   eBook   979-8-89165-178-4
        Paperback   979-8-89165-179-1
        Hardback   979-8-89165-180-7

Cover Design by Abigael Elliott
Interior Layout and Design by Anton Khodakovsky

Published by
STREAMLINE BOOKS
Kansas City, MO
www.streamlinebookspublishing.com

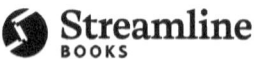

WILL TO LIVE

A Deep Survival Guide to Stage IV Lung Cancer

PAUL D. SEYFERTH

For Jacqulyn

Contents

Advance Praise

....

"As a seasoned radiation oncologist, this book has revitalized my passion for my practice and has added to my desire to be a better patient advocate. If I could, I would ensure that every oncologist today would read this book and add it to their medical library. Using his observational skills, research prowess, and analytical approach, Paul has put together a book that is a must-read for patients facing similar situations."

—KENNETH D. HAUGEN, MD, Radiation Oncology

"A diagnosis of stage IV cancer is a body blow, followed by a round-house punch when the doctor reveals the grim prognosis. That's where survivor Paul Seyferth comes in. An elite courtroom attorney, Seyferth uses his cool analytical mind and his powers of clear communication to produce an invaluable battle plan. No one wants to need this book—but everyone who needs it will be glad that it exists."

—DAVID VON DREHLE, *Washington Post* columnist and author of *The Book of Charlie*

"There is a common denominator amongst cancer survivors who beat the odds—I call it the X factor. The X factor is a mindset; an ethos of resilient hope. Paul possesses the X factor, and this book can help others learn to cultivate it in their own journey to beat the odds."

—LUCAS TIMS, ND, FABNO, Integrative Oncology

"Paul Seyferth set out to write one of those how-to guides, a DIY manual, a 'what to expect when . . .' book—and he did—but the smart reader will also find, among all the advice, an emotionally powerful memoir of a man pioneering at the borderland between death and life."

—JACK HITT, author of *Off the Road: A Modern-Day Walk Down the Pilgrim's Route into Spain*

"*Will to Live* is a powerful and insightful guide for anyone facing a cancer diagnosis, especially those with advanced stages of the disease. Paul D. Seyferth combines his personal experience bringing his encouragement as a survival guide that is both practical and emotionally resonant. Seyferth's emphasis on hope, mental resilience, and personal responsibility in the healing process is particularly compelling. I appreciate his sharing of hope as his testament to the power of determination in facing life with lung cancer."

—TERRI CONNERAN, founder of KRAS Kickers, KRAS Cancer Connect (and seven-plus-year survivor of KRAS-positive lung cancer)

"Paul Seyferth delves into the profound journey of facing cancer—a journey that intertwines the raw challenges of illness with the deep questions of existence. Paul's book is not just a story of survival but a philosophical exploration of what it means to truly live. Through candid reflections, personal stories, and philosophical musings, it offers a roadmap for navigating the emotional and existential terrain that cancer brings. Whether you are a patient, a survivor, or a loved one, Paul invites you to find meaning, strength, and hope in the face of one of life's most daunting challenges. His outlook on how to fight the inner demons is incredibly beneficial, and it translates to other diseases just as easily. A must-read when facing the most frightening parts of life."

"A bobber was once thrown into an angry sea. The waves crashed all around. The wind blew. The bobber hadn't seen this coming. Nor could he see the land from which he had been thrown. In the midst of all those wild distractions, the bobber looked around and saw other bobbers being thrown around in the ocean. He asked, 'How do we get back to land?' The bobbers looked at him with sad eyes and said, 'We can't. We're bobbers. We are at the mercy of the sea, and the wind, and the current. We have no way to swim. Didn't someone tell you that you are a bobber?'

'But what happens to us here?' the bobber asked. Another bobber said, 'This is where we die.'

Our bobber, whose name was Paul Seyferth, decided that being a bobber was a given. But being helpless and hopeless wasn't part of being a bobber. This was a choice. So, Paul said to the other bobbers, 'I may be a bobber, but I don't intend to die here.' And so, he began to experiment. He began to notice how he could use his body to take advantage of the wind and the currents. He heard some bobber say, 'It's a waste of time.' But it wasn't. He learned that the land was far away, but that only increased his resolve. He learned that other bobbers had made it back to land. He decided he would make it back, too.

Paul is standing on the beach. He feels the warm sand on his toes, and the sun gently warms him. He's decided that he'd like other bobbers to know that being a bobber doesn't mean somebody else gets to tell you how you can live. Because Paul learned something really important as he struggled against the currents and the wind and the angry sea. He learned that really living means doing everything you can to make your way back to your wife and daughter, your friends, and those who love you. It means not giving away the precious breath of life without a real fight.

Paul is standing on the beach. You are holding Paul's love story in your hands. 'Come on out,' he's saying to you across the waves and the wind and the current. 'Come on out,' he says, 'the land is just fine.'"

—EDWARD "CHIP" ROBERTSON, former chief justice of the
Missouri Supreme Court

Hope is synonymous with a positive will to live and affects a positive outcome, whatever that might be.

—ERNEST ROSENBAUM, MD, and DAVID SPIEGEL, MD

The will to live is not a will, in the sense of that conscious or 'free will' by which we like to distinguish man from the animal kingdom. It is a biological and psychological force. It is the product of many factors. Like an iceberg which is seven-eighths under water, the will to live is largely submerged below the surface of our consciousness. We can unconsciously weaken and destroy it. But though the will to live is mostly unconscious, it can be strengthened, nourished, cultivated— and this we can do consciously.

—ARNOLD HUTCHISON, MD

Just saying that you want to live is not enough. You must truly want to survive and be willing to do whatever it takes to overcome anything and everything that gets in the way.

—MICHAEL LLOYD

Foreword

BY DR. KENNETH D. HAUGEN

THE BOOK YOU ARE NOW HOLDING IS NOT ONLY AN EFFECTIVE guide for patients with stage IV non-small cell lung cancer but also a much-needed perspective for oncologists around the world. With close to thirty years of experience in radiation oncology, Paul's book has positively affected my medical practice. I believe Paul's insights apply to many other advanced stage cancers and other chronic, life-threatening diseases, providing a useful guide that helps fill a gap in the administration of oncology care.

With my years of experience in my specialty and forty-plus years in health care, I never imagined myself writing the forward of a book about how a close, lifelong friend survived stage IV cancer. I am acutely aware that cancer is nondiscriminatory; however, Paul is one of the last individuals I would have expected to be diagnosed with lung cancer. He has always been the picture of health and discipline, both physically and mentally. To be transparent, when I found out about his diagnosis two years after he began treatments, I was not convinced Paul had been accurately staged. My doubt ultimately led me to have Paul send me a copy of his files, including a disc of his imaging. I personally reviewed his records with a well-respected colleague in the field of radiation oncology. We confirmed, much to my dismay, the accuracy of his diagnosis and stage.

Paul and I have been friends for much of our lives and were particularly close throughout high school. Our unique experiences together have built a special friendship that few are fortunate enough to have. As it turns out, our friendship seems to have been mutually beneficial, each of us attributing much of our success in life to the other. We grew up in a small town in rural Michigan where, after high school, pursuing a trade or working in a local shop was the expectation. Going to college and attending medical school or law school was virtually unheard of.

Paul's father was a well-respected bricklayer and possessed a strong sense of ethics. He demanded excellence from those who worked for him and had little to no patience for incompetence. Though not educated at the collegiate level, I remember Paul's father as quick-witted, intelligent and quite frankly, a somewhat scary man. In turn, Paul experienced a challenging childhood under the influence of his father. When I visited Paul in our high school years, I often found him at his house reading a book while listening to a baseball game, his preferred way of escaping from his challenging family environment. While growing up with Paul, I saw him develop the same strong work ethic and frank honesty as his father. Paul was the first of his family to pursue a university education, and I was not at all surprised as I witnessed his continued success throughout his education and career, where he ultimately became the founder of a very successful law firm in Kansas City.

Our lives eventually took different trajectories, and our interactions became less frequent, dwindling down to updates every two-to-three-years. This is why I didn't hear of my friend's condition until two years after his diagnosis and treatments began. After learning of his diagnosis, I asked Paul why he hadn't let me know sooner, and his answer was simply "I did not want to burden you." I unknowingly had mixed feelings about his decision to not share his burden with me, finding myself more emotional than I expected when I shared the news with my wife. Ironically, because of cancer, our close friendship has rekindled. In our subsequent conversations and meetings since his diagnosis, I have been impressed, but not surprised, by the remarkable insights Paul has gained into all aspects of cancer care. These insights can only be obtained by spending years in the medical profession and/or being an active, analytical participant in one's care as a patient.

Paul's approach to the "mental" side of cancer care, in addition to his description of the complicated dichotomy of the patient/physician relationship, is inspiring. His approach is one that could only be described by someone who has experienced it for themselves. In "typical" Paul fashion, he is not afraid to present the more controversial aspects of cancer care, as is described specifically in the chapters on complementary medicine and the role of a positive mindset. These topics are an ongoing challenge for me and many other oncologists today. Paul's presentation on these complex subjects is supported by research and presented with a balanced approach.

As a seasoned radiation oncologist, this book has revitalized my passion for my practice and has added to my desire to be a better patient advocate. If I could, I would ensure that every practicing oncologist would read this book and add it to their medical library. Using his observational skills, research prowess, and analytical approach, Paul has put together a book that is a must-read for patients facing an advanced cancer diagnosis.

Paul's journey as a cancer survivor over the past five years with stage IV non-small cell lung cancer is a testament to not only my friend's perseverance but also to the care team that he has embraced.

Preface

I REMEMBER THAT IT WAS AN UNUSUALLY COOL AND GRAY SUMMER day the afternoon my wife talked me out of dying.

I was well into my fourth month of chemotherapy and had no less than a couple of additional months of treatments ahead, having been diagnosed with stage IV lung cancer some six months earlier. I had not eaten much in the previous days, had slept only here and there, and my mouth tasted like a sickening combination of fuel oil and metal. I was otherwise feeling comfortable in my "chemo bed," having found something of a sweet spot where nausea seemed to be kept at bay if my head was tilted just right. I hadn't left the bed, except to use the bathroom, in several days. I was drifting in and out of a state between trance and sleep and was getting far too comfortable with the notion that perhaps "my time had come." I was in the twilight of half-surrender, letting myself fade. Fading didn't seem so bad.

My wife, Rebecca, came into the room and sat down next to me by the edge of the bed. She didn't mince words: "Now is not your time to die," she said. "I can see you are fading. Don't go there. We need you to live. You can push through this. Don't you dare get comfortable with dying."

Rebecca has always been able to read me like a book, and she had sensed that I was beginning to close the last chapter of *my* book. She had been suffering just as much as I had, even though she was not the lead actor in this drama. For several months, she and my daughter, Jacqulyn, had valiantly borne the subtle but very real burden of caring for a loved one with cancer.

I listened to and absorbed Rebecca's words. I didn't say much in response, but I knew she was right. I was reminded that I had specifically decided six months earlier to do everything possible to survive, to fight cancer with everything I had. And even in the present condition, I was a blessed man. I was receiving some of the best cancer treatments the world had to offer. I had the loving support of my wife, my daughter, friends, family throughout the country, and even strangers. My condition was objectively improving, but there was no doubt I was losing my resolve. I knew this was a critical moment. My will to live was being tested. That afternoon, Rebecca had called me out and convinced me not to fail this test.

My wife's words marked a turning point. She had said her piece and left the room. That afternoon, I fixed my resolve to continue to live.

The afternoon I have described was over four years ago.

o o o

We really know very little about this mysterious force, the will to live.
—ERNEST H. ROSENBAUM and
ISADORA R. ROSENBAUM, *Inner Fire*

The "will to live" is indeed a mysterious force. One does not usually even contemplate the capacity of marshaling such a force, let alone employing it, absent the adversity inherent in a battle for one's life. This book is about a particularly challenging battle involving what is considered one of the "deadliest" of cancers (i.e., stage IV lung cancer).[1] As such, surviving advanced lung cancer is an almost *perfect* battleground for summoning and then testing one's will to live.

Why do some people survive advanced lung cancer while others do not?

Oncologists have "always been fascinated by the power of the will to live. What makes a person faced with a life-threatening crisis fight to live?"[2] This question is not only an inherent feature of cancer survival but also a throughline in *all* survival settings, such as wilderness accidents, plane crashes, and in response to other deadly diseases. In the words of survival expert Laurence Gonzales, "one of the truly baffling mysteries of 'deep survival' concerns who survives and who doesn't. It's not who you'd predict, either."[3]

Are some people just "lucky"? Is fate involved? Or is there a rhyme or reason behind deep survival? In other words, are there discernable *principles* involved in pushing through a deadly crisis, especially a deadly health crisis?

My answer to this question is the book you hold in your hands. The specific answer to these questions is straightforward: those who *consciously summon, deliberately cultivate,* and *proactively sustain* their will to live have the best chance of surviving advanced lung cancer. Moreover, the fuel for these efforts, and thus the fuel for the will to live, consists of one simple word: *hope.* "Hope keeps one alive to fight another day, a month, a year, and a return to better health."[4]

"Hope as a strategy" for cancer survival sounds like a nice phrase, but how might such a strategy be applied over time and in the trenches for those battling a deadly cancer? My answer to this very practical question is that one's will to live and the hope that fuels it take on different guises as one progresses through the various chronological stages of advanced lung cancer survival.

Initially, the will to live manifests, first and foremost, in a rebellious spirit, the type of spirit that actively responds to the shock of a diagnosis of advanced lung cancer rather than shrinking from it or giving up. This initial phase is the first ninety days after diagnosis, and I call this the phase of *rebellious hope.* After this initial phase, a spirit of rebellious hope is then enhanced and trans-formed by the taking of personal responsibility for one's healing rather than delegating this important task to doctors and others. This second phase is the first year after diagnosis, and I call this the phase of *responsible hope*.

Alas, in too many cases, a spirit of rebelliousness and tak-ing personal responsibility for healing are not enough: because surviving advanced lung cancer is, by definition, a long-term prop-osition, durable resilience is required, as setbacks and obstacles are an almost inherent feature of long-term cancer survival. This third phase encompasses the roughly four-year phase beginning the first year after one's diagnosis (years two through five), and I call this the phase of *resilient hope*. After reaching the five-year survival mark, the durable resilience previously called upon is then enhanced, and one's hope is replenished with the motivation of role models who have survived long-term. This is the long-term phase of lung cancer survival, and I call this the phase of *replen-ished hope*. Finally, throughout all phases of survival, the will to live, that seemingly mysterious arrow in the quiver of long-term survi-vors, must be constantly *rekindled*. This arrow must be deliberately sharpened and then resharpened. This is a daily practice, and I call this all-encompassing phase the phase of *rekindled hope*.

Yes, the will to live is a mysterious force, but I believe that this mystery can be significantly unraveled for the patient with advanced lung cancer, for other types of cancer, for others battling potentially deadly diseases, and for those who find themselves in any "survival" setting. The purpose of this book is to unravel this mysterious force, not just with my thoughts and experiences but with the thoughts and experiences of survival experts, cancer experts, and with the thoughts and experiences of other advanced lung cancer survivors.

"The will to live is in itself an energy," a shorthand for a way of fixing one's resolve, no matter the obstacles.[5] Like other kinds of energy, this energy must first be discovered, tapped into, and then renewed. This renewal may take on different guises, but within these various guises, the bedrock and source of this energy is always hope.

o o o

Several hours after my wife's very direct words on that cool, gray afternoon, I got out of that comfortable bed and hobbled downstairs. Rebecca was staring into the fireplace, lost in thought. She was surprised to see me moving about. I sat down on a couch across from her, vertically upright for the first time in a few days. No profound words were said. I let her know I was hungry and that something like scrambled eggs—one of my three or four food cravings throughout the previous months—sure sounded good. The fog was lifting just a bit.

I then looked at my wife of almost thirty years, the one love of my life, my constant caregiver, and—especially on that memorable afternoon—a world-class deep survival coach, and said the only thing I could think of that made any sense: "Thank you."

INTRODUCTION

People get cancer, and I am one of the people.
>   —MORHAF AL Achkar, MD, PhD, *Roads to Meaning* and
>   *Resilience with Cancer*

Cancer is a mighty blow...especially since it seems to attack indiscriminately. ... Cancer routinely affects those who have no history of illness and have diligently followed the tenants of a healthful life. It's as if the roulette wheel has names in the slots, and a ball called "cancer" bounces randomly until it falls upon some unlucky soul.
>   —C. MICHAEL ARMSTRONG, *Cancer with Hope*

Beginnings

THIS BOOK CANNOT HELP BUT BE SOMETHING OF A PERSONAL memoir.

Let me begin by being quite explicit: there is no magic bullet for surviving advanced lung cancer. The lack of a magic bullet should not blind us, however, to the presence of a sharpened and underused arrow in one's quiver. I have not only sharpened and used that arrow for nearly five years in many different settings but also have read widely and thought deeply about how that arrow has worked for me and how it may work for you.

With that said, I have survived stage IV non-small-cell lung cancer roughly ten times longer than my original prognosis and twice as long as the best-case scenario given by my original oncologist. So, the details of my particular story of survival may be of use to you.

The details I give below are not uncommon among those diagnosed with advanced lung cancer. There is nothing special about my circumstances except, perhaps, that I have lived long enough to write about them. Because I am making some specific suggestions to you in this book for your consideration in dealing with this cancer, and because my suggestions are based upon personal experience, I am going to err on the side of what might be considered too much detail in outlining the details of my survival.*

---

* For those wishing to jump ahead, the appendix contains the Twenty-One "Rules" of Deep Cancer Survival discussed throughout the remainder of the book.

Background

Mid-January of 2020. It had been about two weeks since my life was upended.

In early January, I had been diagnosed with stage IV metastatic non-small-cell lung cancer (NSCLC). While waiting until later in the month to see a lung cancer specialist, I decided that I needed to learn everything possible about the disease that had kicked down the door of an otherwise pleasant life.

I had to learn about this brand-new subject, so I sat down and reviewed books and articles on cancer first, then specifically lung cancer, and then NSCLC. Many books and articles. Movies and videos too. I read nonstop from morning until night for about two weeks, as if cramming for an exam to be given by my not-yet-known oncologist. I read how surprisingly mysterious cancer was. I read about my iteration of the disease—advanced NSCLC, sort of the Honda Accord of cancers. I learned what "metastases" means and why it matters so much. I read claims about miracle remedies involving carrot juice, sauerkraut, Mexican clinics, and even how trampolines might help. I read about survival rates, survival tales, and agonizing deaths. I became something of an amateur statistician.

I read about the wonders and brutal effects of radiation and chemotherapy. I wondered how odd my already too-big head would look without hair. I read about "anti-cancer living," a perfectly useful concept that seemed, in my then-current reading chair, and under the circumstances, more than a day late and more than a dollar short.

I also read polemics on the evils of conventional medical treatments (i.e., Western medicine). I read much about the harms of undergoing and forgoing such conventional medical treatments. I read about how to starve cancer. I read about the evil substance that does just the opposite of starving cancer (short answer: fructose). I read about Otto Warburg and Sydney Farber and learned about cancer whispering and even the best way of "beating crazy odds." I read about mustard gas and apricot seeds. I read and heard about psychics, medical mediums, herbs, acupuncture, the placebo effect, and its less-understood evil twin, the nocebo effect.

I read deeply about autosuggestion (self-hypnosis) and high-dose vitamin treatments. I was even tempted to send twenty-five dollars to that ubiquitous miracle-cure lady whose ad seemingly pops up almost every time anybody Googles something about cancer. I saved that twenty-five dollars and bought another couple of cancer books.

Somewhere in this beginning phase of seeking to understand cancer, my wife and I tried to watch a PBS series on cancer titled *Cancer: The Emperor of All Maladies*. We stopped. It was too depressing. I then became aware that the Pulitzer Prize–winning author of the bestselling book by the same name, who is also an oncologist, had resurrected a catchy, nineteenth-century phrase— "the emperor of all maladies," but was kind enough to leave off the full wording of the phrase in titling his book, the remainder of the phrase that perfectly points out the difference between doctors and their patients (i.e., that cancer may be called the "the emperor of all maladies" but is also "the king of terrors").[6] Cancer is clearly the "emperor of all maladies" if you happen to be an oncologist, but for the newly diagnosed, the phrase "king of terrors" hits much closer to home.

I was also given lots of unsolicited advice by well-meaning family, loved ones, and strangers—lots and lots of it.

One blessing in all of this cramming was that my thirty-plus years as a trial lawyer had equipped me with the mental stamina for the tasks at hand. These included the task of taking in vast amounts of information, picking out the bottom line, sifting through quite a lot of bullshit, mentally cross-examining so-called expert opinions while also digesting such opinions, and most important of all, the task of having to—under fairly strict time constraints—make serious and inherently risky strategic decisions. Seasoned trial lawyers are used to becoming subject-matter experts on a wide array of areas in short bursts of time, but they usually do so with *other* people's lives and money at stake. Here, the decisions to be made involved *my* life and the life of my family, so—for those few weeks—I was in "trial prep" overload.

You will hear about the decisions I made below, decisions that were a combination of rational analysis, intuitive recognition, and, yes, even luck. Thankfully, and given the stacked odds in play, the most important of those decisions have seemed to turn out "right."

Almost the entire time I was searching and reading and reading and searching, I couldn't help but wonder: Why has nobody written a comprehensive book for the person in my shoes, dealing with essentially the deadliest and most commonly diagnosed form of cancer? Where was the book that specifically addressed advanced lung cancer for the person needing to make life-altering decisions about brutally difficult treatment options, all while staring the prospect of not-too-distant death in the face? Where was the book for the anguished loved ones helplessly looking on while this process unfolded?

When Rebecca was pregnant in 2000, nearly every soon-to-be parent we knew could buy and read a book about "what to expect when you're expecting." We bought one immediately once we found out Rebecca was pregnant, and it was a critical handbook for one of life's major challenges. The book was not only an orientation but also something of a road map.

Where was that same type of book for those diagnosed with advanced lung cancer?

Somewhere in that haze of those weeks of nonstop reading and obsessing, I decided that when I survived what loomed ahead, I would write the book I was then looking for and not finding. The book would be my best judgment about how to survive some seriously choppy skies in a plane with a too-high probability of crashing. The book would combine "theory" and "practice," and it might also have the credibility that attaches when someone puts their money where their mouth is (i.e., when the strategies and the courses of action suggested have actually resulted in a statistically unexpected survival).

How cool would that be, I fantasized, highlighter in hand, brain in high gear, staring at that stack of dog-eared books.

o o o

Let me again be quite explicit: I know exactly how you feel right now. Your world has been turned upside down. You are overwhelmed. Your family is overwhelmed. Nobody plans for a "terminal" cancer diagnosis.

Likewise, nobody prepares in advance for how to *respond* once such a diagnosis breaks into one's life. You and I are truly comrades in the way that people become comrades in almost every deadly survival setting. It is my firm belief that those who have been through the plane crash can truly help others in the same position. In this sense, we are comrades in arms, fellow passengers on the plane, a plane that has been invaded by a deadly hijacker. Action is required, and there is no time to waste. In the words of Laurence Gonzalez, the "first role is to face reality. Good survivors aren't immune to fear. They know what's happening, and it does 'scare the living shit out of them.' It's all a question of what you do next."[7]

My hope is that what follows helps you and your loved ones gain some peace of mind and the tools to survive advanced lung cancer. I am offering you some hard-earned lessons about *what to do next*. I am not offering you medical advice, but I do offer something equally important: survival advice.

If the premise of this book is sound, there is something akin to a set of "skills" that allows one to maximize the chances of surviving advanced-stage lung cancer. The core *skill* involves an unbridled focus on one of the few areas in which a cancer survivor has a modicum of control (i.e., the "mental" side of cancer survival), sometimes described as a way to "turn on our bodies' own incredible self-healing capabilities."[8] The core *strategy* of this mental game is the intentional, thoughtful, and persistent rekindling of the will to live, the core *fuel* for this strategy is hope, and the core *tactics* for implementing this strategy constitute the remaining portions of this book.

Before we dive into this strategy and its related tactics, let me give you some details about my treatment history and the structure of the remainder of this book.

Treatment Background and Medical History

As I finish the final draft of this book, I am what cancer researcher and author Kelly Turner would call a "Radical Remission" cancer survivor, a survivor whose remission is "statistically unexpected."[9] As I am finalizing the draft of this book, my five-year anniversary from the date of my original diagnosis looms in a few days. I also fall into the type of Radical Remission category described by Turner as a cancer patient "[who] uses conventional and alternative healing methods at the same time in order to outlive a statistically dire prognosis (i.e., any cancer with a less than 25 percent chance of five-year survival)."[10] Such individuals are also described as "exceptional responders."[11]

As I have mentioned, I was diagnosed with stage IV-NSCLC in January 2020, just a few weeks before the worldwide COVID pandemic. I was then fifty-seven years old, a husband to an amazing wife of twenty-nine years, and the father of a thriving eighteen-year-old daughter. I had spent thirty-three years as a trial lawyer with a successful law firm I founded in 2003. I had reached nearly every goal I had set out to attain as a trial lawyer. Life was "very good" for our family and for me. Prior to my diagnosis, I had decided to step away from the rigors of over three decades of litigation work and had completed an application to become a trial judge. My plan was to voluntarily walk away from a successful career and dedicate myself to public service as a judge. Many of the harshest of life's struggles—and like everybody reading this book, there had been more than a few—seemed to be in the rearview mirror.

As is so common with an NSCLC diagnosis, "out of nowhere," I began experiencing symptoms of a heavy cough and severe fatigue over the Thanksgiving weekend of 2019. I was initially diagnosed by my primary physician with pneumonia, which, after a couple of weeks, was "upgraded" to double pneumonia and then upgraded to a collapsed lung. By mid-December, I was getting no better with antibiotics and was referred to a pulmonologist, where a CT scan was ordered. The CT scan showed something in my right lung concerning enough that a PET scan was ordered for late December 2019. The results of the PET scan were not good, nor was the outcome of a subsequent biopsy. I had a tumor of approximately 2.5 by 2.0 centimeters in my right lung, which had spread to my lymph nodes and the T6 vertebra in my spine.

I was diagnosed by my then and current oncologist with adenocarcinoma, stage IV NSCLC. Like so many other advanced cancer patients who receive this diagnosis, the question was asked: "How long have I got?" I was told that, without effective treatment, I had four to six months to live. The best-case scenario with effective treatment was two years. I was given this prognosis one day before I was supposed to turn in an application to become a trial judge.

I never turned in the judicial application.

∘ ∘ ∘

Prior to all of this, I was a generally healthy person.

I did not smoke. As of January 2020, I had not had a drop of alcohol in fourteen months. I exercised regularly and, in my early fifties, obtained a first and then second-degree black belt in Okinawan karate. I competed in amateur golf tournaments around the country and even competed in a senior national championship.

Although I carried around ten to twenty unwanted pounds at any given time, I had been told by my doctor throughout my fifties that I was usually the "healthiest person" he had seen on that particular day, and I believed him. My "life force" felt great. Diseases were something other people experienced—not me.

I felt invulnerable, physically, prior to the strange year of 2020.

I suspect some version of this story is common to those with a late-stage lung cancer diagnosis. The diagnosis truly does seem to come from the blind side.

As the quotes at the beginning of this book demonstrate, the *psychological* component of the diagnosis cannot be underestimated. It is one thing to hear tales of others who have had their "world turned upside down." It is quite another to experience this firsthand—while also being confronted by the prospect of one's potentially imminent death. Yes, I clearly understand and then understood that we are *all* going to die someday. Usually, however, one is not put "on the clock" quite so abruptly, nor is one usually put "on the clock" and *then* told that what time remains on that clock will consist of a series of poisonings, sickness, and severe disruption.

A quite apt cliché about cancer is that the "cancer club" is not a club anybody ever seeks to join. Like any restricted-membership club, those who have joined seemed to have a certain understanding of one another. Embedded within that tacit understanding for those with advanced cancer is a shared experience—the shared experience of having one's world turned upside down while *also* seriously confronting, perhaps for the first time, the prospect of one's rapidly approaching death. Not to put too fine a point on it, but those not a part of this "club" cannot truly understand this.

I was completely oblivious to this understanding, even when my friend Mark went through a "stage four" cancer experience ten years before my diagnosis. Mark was one of the first persons I told of my diagnosis. The look on his face said it all. Mark, a decorated Vietnam veteran, a ten-year survivor of stage IV esophageal cancer, a mentor, and one of my best friends, happened to be in my office the day or two after my diagnosis. He took a brief look at my PET scan summary, looked me straight in the eye, and in his quiet, powerful, and understated way, said, "Paul, your situation is very grave." This shook me more than anything a doctor has ever told me.

Let's face it: if you are a member of the advanced-stage lung cancer club, your situation is also very grave. You are likely going to need some very powerful and toxic treatments as soon as possible. But you are also going to need to learn how to "treat" yourself, as well.

○ ○ ○

One of the unfortunate elements of the cancer world in the present day is, in my opinion, the false dichotomy between "orthodox" and "alternative" cancer treatment modalities. For the more curious of those diagnosed with any form of cancer, this dichotomy becomes readily apparent as one begins assessing treatment options.

Not long after my diagnosis, I quickly determined that this seeming dichotomy needed to be rejected. Instead, I determined early on to employ what I call a "parallel silo" approach to cancer treatments. Each treatment I reviewed and then undertook would be viewed within its own silo, and my goal would be to utilize as many *parallel* treatment silos as possible, so long as they did not conflict or lessen the effectiveness of any other given treatment. To illustrate, one of my early oncologists supported the idea of my doing acupuncture in conjunction with my chemotherapy treatments, but she did not think it wise to take Chinese herbs while undergoing those treatments. She was concerned about the interaction between the herbs and the chemotherapy drugs: two different treatment paradigms but with a minimal chance of them working against each other. As you will learn further in this book, I pursued the "parallel silo" approach in many different ways over the past five years.

For now, I think it important to lay out the basic outline of the orthodox medical treatments I have undertaken since January 2020. Within weeks of my initial diagnosis, I obtained a second opinion at one of the premier cancer treatment centers, MD Anderson Cancer Center, in Houston, Texas. This second opinion confirmed the initial diagnosis, but my MD Anderson oncologist dramatically altered the proposed treatment plan I had originally been given. Thankfully, my local Kansas City oncologist did not harbor professional pride or other considerations that might get in the way, and he was able to execute the second-opinion treatment plan with alacrity.

That first phase of treatments, within the first ninety days after diagnosis, consisted of fifteen daily radiation treatments to the tumor in my right lung in February and March of 2020, a time frame that unfortunately coincided with the worldwide COVID pandemic. In April of 2020, I then began eighteen weeks of chemotherapy, administered once every three weeks. The chemotherapy combination was carboplatin, Alimta, and Avastin. After that four-to-five-month phase, I then went on "maintenance" chemotherapy with Avastin alone for another three to four months until near the end of 2020, at which time I decided to halt the maintenance program because of overall toxicity, fatigue, and generally positive scans.

This was the orthodox treatment plan I pursued in the first year after diagnosis. After that first year, I was wiped out. As I alluded to earlier, the treatments came close to killing me.

Another recurring theme of this book is that you must take responsibility for your situation. One way this occurs is by learning about your disease or by becoming what survivor Glenn Sabin calls a "citizen-scientist."[12] Throughout the course of the last five years, and even while suffering the worst of the effects of treatments, I tried to stay abreast of scientific and medical studies related to lung cancer and cancer in general. I have become something of a "lay expert" on NSCLC, the kind of patient some oncologists find quite annoying.

In pursuit of my "parallel silo" approach, I aggressively pursued complementary treatments while undergoing chemotherapy. By way of example, and as discussed in a separate chapter below, I have received regular treatments of high-dose vitamin C, and I have also received regular treatments for acupuncture as well. These were provided by cancer specialists in both areas.

But I learned that one must also push the envelope with what are considered orthodox treatments as well. As one example of this, in late 2020, I came across a study that indicated that the damage done to lung tissue by radiation could be repaired by a regimen of hyperbaric oxygen therapy. After getting a referral from my oncologist in February 2021, the director of wound care at the local University of Kansas Health System put me on a forty-day regimen of hyperbaric oxygen treatments (HBO2), which consisted of daily two-hour sessions within the equivalent of an oversized glass coffin, while purified oxygen was pumped into my healing lungs. I do not know whether HBO2 *healed* my lungs, but it certainly seemed to put me back on my feet after the year of treatments I have described above.

All in all, about a year after my initial diagnosis, life seemed to be getting back on track. Throughout the previous year of treatment, I had remained active. I had played golf at least once a week, stayed social, and kept a pretty vigorous reading pace both in the cancer world and other areas of interest. I had also kept up a decent output of watercolor paintings, a hobby I had started around 2007. I had even begun writing this book.

Then, just as things were starting to look up, I was diagnosed with prostate cancer. Ironically, the indications of prostate cancer seeped into a PET scan I had been given in the summer of 2021, and were thus caught fairly early.

At first, my lung oncologist didn't seem all that concerned about the indications of potential prostate cancer and even suggested that follow-up was unnecessary. Thankfully, Rebecca thought otherwise. After several tests and a biopsy, I was diagnosed with adenocarcinoma in my prostate, with what is called a "favorable intermediate" diagnosis. Prostate cancer is not "staged" like lung cancer, but this diagnosis was roughly the equivalent of a stage IIa NSCLC diagnosis.

After much further reading and strategizing and on doctor's advice, I decided against the orthodox trio of typical prostate cancer treatments (radiation, surgery, or "wait and see"). Instead, I traveled in February 2022 to south Florida to have a "laser ablation" procedure performed on the prostate cancer. I have described this as a very expensive (not covered by insurance) type of spot-welding of my prostate cancer. The spot-welding worked. The laser ablation was "successful." Was the month-long catheter painful? Yes. And so was the bill. But my prostate cancer was (and is) at bay. By around February of 2022—fully almost twenty-four months after my initial stage IV NSCLS diagnosis—I was a bona fide two-time cancer survivor, feeling pretty good, and about to outlast the original "best-case scenario."

This welcome and well-earned respite would last for about three or four months.

In the late summer of 2022, a CT scan revealed that a couple of my originally affected lymph nodes were swollen. Thereafter, a PET scan was performed, and it turned out that several of the originally cancerous lymph nodes "lit up"—never a good sign—as well as the original spot on my spine. There was also a new spot of concern on my *left* lung, which had seemingly never been present before. Thirty-two months after my initial lung cancer diagnosis and several months after dealing with an independent prostate cancer diagnosis, I had a bona fide lung cancer recurrence. The original cancer had returned, with a possible bonus lesion in my left lung.

I again sought a second opinion on treatment from my original second-opinion oncologist at MD Anderson, and I was back in chemotherapy by September 2022. This would be the same as my original regimen. I did four cycles of this same chemotherapy. These treatments were as brutal as the first go-around, if not worse. Nevertheless, the treatments were effective. After a scan revealed positive progress, my treatments then converted over to radiation ablation. This radiation ablation consisted of twenty days of radiation in which five different spots in my torso were radiated to the tune of about one hour per day. That radiation ended in mid-February 2023, more than three years after my initial diagnosis. The radiation and its effects were brutal as well, and I now have a series of tattoos on various parts of my body as a lifelong reminder of the experience.

As I write this book, I have received an excellent PET scan result in June 2023 and "clean" confirmatory CT scans for almost a year. My energy is getting better, and I am golfing, reading, painting, and have (finally) finished this book. In November of 2023, I also received a clean confirmatory MRI related to my prostate cancer and have suffered no long-term side effects from having had prostate cancer.

It is technically true that I am a multiple-cancer survivor and have "beaten" cancer not just once or twice but arguably three different times. It is more accurate to say, however, that I am "alive with disease." AWD is the acronym used in the stage IV lung cancer world. Not a very inspiring term, but accurate nonetheless. Very early on, I was told by my MD Anderson oncologist that there is no "cure" for stage IV NSCLC. Because there is no cure, AWD is the best one can hope for—a transition from having what some call a "terminal" disease to instead having a chronic disease. The challenge, every single day, is to extend that window of being AWD.

I have joked with family and friends that my goal in surviving cancer is hopefully to someday die of something else, preferably quite suddenly. Right now, I am on track for that goal.

o o o

One reason I have shared this treatment summary with you in some detail is so that you may see that I have great confidence in modern orthodox cancer treatments. After all, I have spent the better part of a year in first-line and maintenance chemotherapy. Likewise, I have spent seven full weeks in intense radiation therapy on at least five different parts of my body. I have felt the notorious brunt of these treatments too. There have been times when I have gone close to a week without eating. I have spent holidays in the local emergency room, bleeding from places not usually discussed in polite society. I could describe additional unpleasant side effects—effects I experience on a daily basis—but you get the point.

I do not minimize the brutality of traditional cancer treatments. But I do not minimize their effectiveness either. Indeed, I would likely have had prostate surgery—and thus completed the "oncology trifecta" of radiation, chemotherapy, and surgery—had not the novel treatment of laser ablation come to my attention.

When it comes to cancer treatments, I have seen and felt it all and have ridden the roller coaster experienced by many of you reading this book. More importantly, I have survived to talk and write about it.

The Structure of This Book

THE STRUCTURE OF THIS BOOK IS DRIVEN BY THE FOLLOWING question, alluded to in the preface: Are there particular chronological time frames that make the most sense in a discussion of surviving advanced lung cancer, and in particular NSCLC? [Throughout the remainder of these pages, I will be focusing on my particular iteration of lung cancer, stage IV NSCLC]. When one is first diagnosed, one hears of "five-year survival rates" and other types of percentages without necessary context. We are going to avoid these types of general discussions in this book, and we are going to be fairly specific about the various courses of action as they relate to the distinct time frames for survival.

Advanced NSCLC survival can be broken down into very specific and scientifically accepted time frames. Although I didn't know about such time frames until I began writing this book, it turns out that the worldwide prevalence of NSCLC allows the person diagnosed to view, with some strong predictive value, the chronological "phases" of advanced NSCLC survival. Before discussing these specific phases, however, let's first examine the prevalence of advanced NSCLC in the context of cancer as a whole.

In 2024, the year of this book's publishing, it is a safe assumption that there will be approximately one million new cases of stage IV NSCLC lung cancer diagnosed worldwide. This may seem like an awfully precise prediction, but the history of the incidence of advanced NSCLC is well-documented.

Advanced NSCLC breaks down as follows on an annual, world-wide basis: in 2020, there were an estimated eighteen million new cancer cases around the world; these eighteen million cases involved every type of the almost two hundred different kinds of cancer. Two million of those new cases were lung cancer (that is, approximately 12 percent of all new cancer cases worldwide specifically involved *lung cancers*). Of those 12 percent of new lung cancer cases, roughly 1.6 million of the two million new cases were NSCLC (i.e., 80 percent of all diagnosed lung cancers are NSCLC lung cancers). Most of the 1.6 million newly diagnosed NSCLC cases in 2020 were *advanced* lung cancers, having spread and metastasized to other parts of the body, and *stage IV* NSCLC cases accounted for more than 50 percent of *all* NSCLC cases. Thus, approximately 800,000 of the 18 million cases of new cancers worldwide were advanced stage IV NSCLC.

Put a different way, in 2020, *roughly 6 percent of all new cancers worldwide were cases of stage IV NSCLC.* Of the two hundred different types of cancers—from stage 0 melanoma to childhood cancers to every stage of breast or prostate cancer—six of one hundred of those cancers were stage IV NSCLC. Please do not gloss over these figures. These are truly almost mind-boggling numbers, and remember: these figures do not include stage III NSCLC, or other advanced lung cancer pathologies.

In the so-called war on cancer, lung cancer generally and advanced stage NSCLC specifically are most assuredly the "front line," where the largest concentration of troops is gathered. No other type of cancer really comes close. And no other type of cancer racks up anywhere near the casualties. Advanced NSCLC is thus among the most statistically significant battles in the war on cancer and one of the deadliest.[13]

o o o

The prevalence of stage IV NSCLC and the statistics I have referred to above are well-documented in a state-of-the-art discussion of 2020 NSCLC cases published in a peer-reviewed study in late 2021, which I have already referred to as the 2020 NSCLC Study. Because that study directly relates to the chronological time frames for viewing long-term survival and the structure of this book and is otherwise central to some of the themes in this book, it is worthy of some detailed discussion.

In late 2021, a nice round-numbered sample of roughly one thousand NSCLC-stage IV patients was the subject of the 2020 NSCLC Study.[14] In that study, titled *How Long Have I Got*, the researchers set out to track the survival rates of those diagnosed with stage IV NSCLC in order to determine what might allow oncologists to answer the question most often asked by advanced NSCLC patients: "How long have I got?" In seeking to answer this question, the authors conducted what appears to be the most current research regarding survival rates for stage IV NSCLC. The researchers came to a number of remarkable conclusions.

Initially, the researchers found that, of the roughly one thousand persons diagnosed with stage IV NSCLC, only 70 percent survived beyond the first three months after diagnosis. In the understated words of the study, "Most lung cancer patients worldwide [stage IV (NSCLC)] have a poor survival: 25–30% die <3 months."[15] This specific figure is worth focusing on for a moment: of those who have been newly diagnosed with stage IV NSCLC, according to the findings of the 2020 NSCLC study, *statistically speaking*, roughly 70 percent of that patient population will live more than three months. We will discuss how to assess survival rates in a coming chapter, but thankfully, you—the reader of this book—are not a statistic. You are literally an "n of 1." Nevertheless, this survival rate is, on its surface, rather sobering news. On an annualized basis, the survival rate for the three months after diagnosis is indeed very poor.

After reviewing the first ninety days after diagnosis, the authors of the study then used additional chronological time frames to assess survival rates among the stage IV NSCLC population. Having begun with the ninety-day window we have just discussed, which I refer to in this book as Phase One, the researchers then assessed survival rates for the remaining nine months after the first year after diagnosis. The survival rates for these remaining nine months of Phase Two increased rather dramatically, as is discussed further in an upcoming chapter. Throughout this book, I have termed that nine-month time frame as Phase Two. After the one-year mark, the authors then assessed survival rates for a three-year period between years two and five after diagnosis, which, in this book, I have referred to as Phase Three. Again, finally, the researchers addressed survival rates for the general time frame, including years five through ten, which I have termed Phase Four.

o o o

These distinct phases related to long-term advanced NSCLC survival provide a useful paradigm for the organization of this book. The structure of this book thus tracks the various phases of advanced NSCLC survival outlined in the 2020 Study. The strategies and issues I discuss must, by necessity, be presented chronologically in this sense, but this breakdown into various phases of NSCLC is nothing more than a conceptual construct. There is no objectively rigorous timing for addressing the strategies and issues presented below. The cancer patient with a stage IV diagnosis is best served by considering *all* the information presented below and then determining the best timing and implementation of which, if any, are undertaken.

Part I of this book is specifically focused on Phase One, the initial ninety-day window after a stage IV NSCLC diagnosis. In part I, *rebellious hope* is, in my opinion, the most essential element to cancer survival. The subjects addressed in Phase One are specifically tailored to help you with surviving these first ninety days and introduce you to the central theme of this book, that it is the "will to live" that helps to explain why some people survive long-term and others do not. You will note that nearly every chapter in the remainder of this book takes the form of an *active* course of action on your part. The table of contents can be viewed as something like a checklist of actions for you to contemplate and then execute, depending upon where you are chronologically in surviving cancer.

Part I is, in many ways, the most important part of this book, not only because of the seemingly dire statistics I have referenced above but also because the newly-diagnosed cancer patient is often drowning in advice, information, and other sources of information likely to cause a sense of overwhelm, and must do so in the face of a not-too-distant and not-improbable prospect of death. This is, to put it mildly, a lot to juggle. There is no sugarcoating the importance of the first ninety days after diagnosis. The 2020 study reaches some distinct conclusions about survival during Phase I, and we will discuss those findings throughout part I. Part I is my attempt to introduce you to the concept of "will to live," to help you approach the issue of survival in the first ninety days, and to prepare you for the challenges ahead.

Part II of this book focuses on the first year after a stage IV NSCLC diagnosis and assumes, obviously, that you have successfully navigated the first ninety days after diagnosis. In part II,

we will see that if the will to live is to become a paramount factor in surviving long-term, this requires the taking of personal
responsibility for your healing. Part II is also a little less theoretical than part I. The dust has settled at least a little bit, and it is
now time to start counterpunching, so to speak. Although there
is no single "open sesame" for every single NSCLC patient, part
II addresses recurring themes in cancer survival and introduces
some mental strategies necessary for navigating the first year
after diagnosis.

Part III focuses on the two-to-five-year mark after a stage IV
NSCLC diagnosis. Here, I contend that the way the will to live is
manifested is by the term *resilience*. This is the middle phase of the
"long haul" of surviving advanced lung cancer. Here, some of the
survival skills addressed in parts I and II will need to be refined
and expanded.

Part IV focuses on the five-to-ten-year mark after a stage IV
NSCLC diagnosis and provides the stories of role models who are
long-term survivors of advanced lung cancer. Phase IV focuses
on the actual long haul, which, as I have mentioned, has been
awkwardly described as "AWD." In this part of the book, I have collected seven publicly available survivor stories of those who lived
five to ten years past their diagnosis of advanced lung cancer and,
where possible, interviewed them to hear their explanation of
how they survived. I have searched for and interviewed the plane
crash survivors, in other words.

Part V is a discussion, in some depth, of a significant self-healing strategy I have pursued over the past five years, a daily strategy
for the rekindling of hope and, thus, the will to live. Part V introduces a conscious, purposeful method of sharpening the arrow in
one's healing quiver we are calling the will to live. The strategy I
present in part V can be implemented by you right now. Other than

my personal circumstances or on my recommendation within my circle of cancer friends and acquaintances, I am not aware of this strategy being described or implemented by any other person fighting cancer. Part V presents a strategy for self-healing that might be pursued by *anybody* with a disease, whether breast cancer, prostate cancer, or heart disease.

Part V is an introduction to a healing strategy called "autosuggestion." Autosuggestion is sometimes called self-hypnosis. The method of autosuggestion I describe in part V and immediately adopted in early 2020—even before I was "officially" diagnosed—was pioneered by a French hypnotist, Émile Coué, in the late 1800s. I have termed this method the Émile Coué method (ECM) and have used the ECM method of autosuggestion twice daily since January 2020. The ECM is quite simple: it calls for you to recite the following suggestion twenty times in the morning and twenty times in the evening in the period of transition between sleep and wakefulness: "Every day, in every way, I am getting better and better." The ECM takes about five minutes per day.

I will describe the ECM in further detail in part V. And for what it's worth, I have recited this suggestion under the conditions suggested by Coué somewhere in the neighborhood seventy thousand times since I was diagnosed.

o o o

The basic message of this book has gone through several iterations.

My first thought was to write a comprehensive handbook, as I have described above. At another point, I tried to gather the stories of a hundred survivors of stage IV lung cancer. As I progressed further with this strategy, however, it became obvious that something more like my original idea of a handbook was called for, with a focus on the mental game of cancer survival, tied to chronological phases. Ultimately, after many fits and starts and several intervening cancers and cancer treatments, I decided to focus thematically on the importance of that mysterious force called the will to live.

The result of my research, my own experience in surviving stage IV lung cancer, and the collected wisdom of other long-term survivors can now, perhaps, be a beginning to the writing of *your* story of survival and your particular handbook for survival.

PART I

Rebellious Hope and the First Ninety Days

Psychologists who study survival say that people who are rule followers don't do as well as those who are of independent mind and spirit. When a patient is told he has six months to live, he has two choices: to accept the news and die, or to rebel and live. People who survive in the face of such a diagnosis are notorious.

—LAURENCE GONZALES, *Deep Survival: Who Lives, Who Dies, and Why*

Radical Remission survivors are the "annoying" patients who do not automatically do whatever their doctors tell them to do.... They are car fanatics who research the best fuel and motor oil, clean and wax their cars regularly, and never miss an oil change. When it comes to their health, they take a very active role in the healing process.

—KELLY TURNER, *Radical Remission: Surviving Cancer Against All Odds*

Chapter 1: *Understanding the Importance of Rebellious Hope*

We all need to find the light in rebellious hope, to keep the flame burning in our darkest hours.

—Dame Deborah James

In this book, the first ninety days after diagnosis are referred to as Phase One of your survival.

If you are a stage IV NSCLC or similarly staged lung cancer patient, there is a strong likelihood that you have been told or have otherwise learned in Phase One that your cancer is "incurable," that you have a short time to live, or that there is not much you can do about this. You may have even repeated these words to others when asked about your condition. These are just a few of the core notions that make up conventional wisdom about advanced lung cancer. By the end of part I, my hope is that you will have seen that these notions, and any words alluding to such notions, must be eliminated from your cancer vocabulary.

Rebellious hope is a pushing against what is considered conventional wisdom. Put another way, what will help you in your darkest hours is the rejection of so-called conventional wisdom about your condition. This constitutes the core element of rebellion during Phase One.

What does this mean?

Laurence Gonzales states this matter very starkly in the book I have quoted in previous pages: "When a patient is told that he has six months to live, he has two choices: to accept the news and die, or to rebel and live. People who survive in the face of such a diagnosis are notorious."[16] "Rebel and live" is Gonzalez's description of notorious survivors. I call this *rebellious hope*. The initial element of rebellious hope is understanding the role *you* play in your survival. You are not a bystander but an active participant, in that survival. Gonzales emphasizes that "scientists have long observed the seeming mystery: You can will yourself to die."[17] But—and this is the core question presented in this book—can you will yourself to live?

The answer is yes: There is a will to live and also a will to die.[18]

The first act of rebellious hope is thus the realization that you—the recently diagnosed cancer patient—have far more agency over your survival than you can imagine right now. You must push against the notion that you have little or no role in your survival.

In the building where I have received the vast number of cancer treatments I have described, one cannot walk through the doors without seeing the names of the cancer center's two generous benefactors: Annette and Rich Bloch. Richard Bloch survived over twenty years past his advanced-stage lung cancer diagnosis and then died of other health conditions. The Blochs' generosity toward others with cancer is a continuing gift to the Kansas City community and communities throughout the United States. A less well-known fact about the Blochs is that they have also written extensively about surviving cancer. In one of their books, *Fighting Cancer*, they state: "The will to live is in itself an energy. It is a desire to fight for life because there is honestly something to live for. The shock and uncertainty of diagnosis cause many people to lose this and suspend living for a few weeks."[19]

Paradoxically, it is right after diagnosis that the will to live is required most. In their book, written in the 1980s, the Blochs quote an unnamed doctor whose comments about various types of cancer patients are quite profound: the doctor stated, "About 15 to 20 percent of people who are seriously ill would prefer to die if given the opportunity, 50 to 60 percent are willing to get better so long as the doctor does the work and the medicine doesn't taste too bad. The final 15–20 percent say, *'I'll do anything I have to do to get well. Just show me'*"[20] (emphasis added). The Blochs further quote this same doctor at some length: "There is no such thing as false hope…it's never therapy that heals, it's people who heal, and the best role for doctors is to encourage that healing process, to help some of the 50 to 60 percent who want the doctor to do all the work *to move over to the realm of survivors*"[21] (emphasis added).

The first printing of *Fighting Cancer* was in 1985. Now, some forty years later, cancer survival has in some ways progressed, but the paradigm described above and the importance of the will to live have not changed.

The first lesson here in Phase One? *You* possess the capacity to "move over to the realm of survivors."

o o o

The second element of the conventional wisdom about advanced NSCLC that must be rejected is the notion that NSCLC—or any other type of cancer diagnosis—is somehow uniquely *incurable*. I have met cancer patients in several different contexts who mention that "my cancer is uncurable," or words to this effect. This is sometimes said with an air of futility, as though such people face an almost impossible uphill fight in the survival process.

You will recall that my MD Anderson doctor made a very specific point to make sure I understood that stage IV NSCLC is presently incurable. What she failed to mention, however, is the very relevant broader context that *no cancer* is "curable." Why does this seemingly pessimistic additional context matter? It matters because, until an actual cure is found for cancer generally, there is no specific significance that attaches to the fact that advanced lung cancer—just like every other cancer—is, at the present time, incurable. And yet, we all know many, many people who have lived long lives with a wide array of various cancers. "'Cures' exist for only a tiny fraction of cancer patients."[22] Unfortunately, this is not likely to change any time soon. "Five decades into the war on cancer it seems clear that no single 'cure' is likely to be forthcoming."[23]

There is nothing unique about the incurability of advanced NSCLC, as compared to virtually every other type of cancer, multiple sclerosis, muscular dystrophy, or most coronary diseases. As with many of these various cancers, we all know people who have lived long lives with these incurable but chronic conditions as well. In Phase One and beyond, it is important for you to set your determination to become one of these survivors. Realizing this fundamental fact about the state of cancer generally *and placing it in its proper context* takes the sting out of your having been diagnosed with advanced lung cancer, does it not?

This Phase One realization is an act of hopeful rebellion because it is the turning of conventional wisdom on its head; this understanding converts what is portrayed as an ostensibly incurable condition into a chronic condition to manage until a cure is discovered.

o o o

The same core principle—the spirit of pushing against—applies to the third element of conventional wisdom about advanced NSCLC or other lung cancer: discussions of prognosis or "how long" you will live.

It is important that you understand what follows and understand it deeply at the core of your being: *nobody* knows how long you have to live, nor does anybody have any business *telling you* how long you have to live. You must *reject* and rebel against anything any doctor or anybody else tells you about your prognosis, or "how long" *you*—the person reading this book—will live. Whether you are polite or annoying in this act of rebellion is up to you, but you should not countenance any such predictions.

This kind of rebellious hope is exemplified by long-term survivor Rick Fields, who is featured in the Rosenbaums' book *Inner Fire: Your Will To Live: Stories of Courage, Hope and Determination.*[24] He was given some version of the usual prognosis after being diagnosed with advanced lung cancer. In *Inner Fire*, he describes his response: "I told one of my doctors, 'You are also going to live until you die. You think you know when I'm going to die. You don't even know when you yourself are going to die.'"[25] He then states, "My first response was definitely a warrior energy toward this cancer which I felt I had to fight."[26] *Warrior energy.* I love that term. It is a term every cancer survivor must learn to be comfortable with, appreciate, and consider cultivating in Phase One.

I was in a similar situation to Rick Fields in January 2020. Remember: I had been cramming for a couple of weeks. I suspected some discussion of prognosis would probably occur. As I have described, after being formally diagnosed, my oncologist informed me—in the presence of my wife—that my prognosis was four to six months without effective treatment and two years as a best-case scenario.

There was a stunned silence after these comments. Rebecca was in shock. I looked at my doctor very directly and simply said, "I reject that." I then asked him the equivalent of the question I had been asked by so many new clients about an upcoming trial: "How many cases like this have you won?" I asked him, in effect, how many of his prior patients had "run the table" on stage IV NSCLC.

His answer was that a couple had survived long-term. I felt some of the warrior energy described by Rick Fields and responded, "Well, Doctor, we're about to get your numbers up."

After this meeting, on the ride home, I emphasized to my distraught wife that we must ignore what we had just heard. "Don't let it be a hex. There is a trap here. Don't fall into that trap. I reject that trap. You should too." I was basing my tough talk in the above meeting on my intuition that I would survive and my decision that I would fight for that survival however I possibly could.

At the time these statements were made, I had not heard of Rick Fields. The 2020 NSCLC study had not yet commenced. But *you* now know *why* such talk should be rejected. At every critical juncture along the path of surviving NSCLC, you have every opportunity to be one of those who survive, whether that is in Phases One, Two, Three or Four. Any discussion of a general prognosis or what the averages say is literally not relevant to your specific survival.

Yes, my dear friend Mark was correct in my office that day: my situation, as is yours in Phase One, was indeed "very grave." I am not suggesting that you engage in denial about this. If you haven't yet decided to do so, however, it is *now* time for you too to rebel in the face of the situation in which you now find yourself. This means turning conventional wisdom on its head.

"Rebellious hope" does not ensure your survival, but as Dame Deborah—the person who seems to have coined this wonderful term—has said, this will "keep the flame burning in our darkest hours."

Chapter 2: *Crossing the Rubicon—The Decision to Fight*

We often ask our patients to explain how they are able to transcend their problems. We have found however diverse they are in ethnic or cultural background, age, educational level, or type of illness ... they have all gone through a similar process of psychological recovery. They all made a "decision to live."

ERNEST AND ISADORA ROSENBAUM, "The Will to Live,"
Stanford Medicine

I AM GOING TO ASSUME YOU NOW APPRECIATE THE NEED TO REBEL against conventional wisdom about lung cancer survival. With that assumption in place, how else does one *become* the type of "notorious" cancer survivor referred to by Laurence Gonzales? Advanced lung cancer survivor Michael Lloyd puts it this way: "The first and most important step in surviving cancer is to decide you want to live."[27]

Let's start from the beginning: you have just come home from the meeting with your oncologist. She has explained to you that your diagnosis is stage IV NSCLS. She pointed out some smoky smears on your CT scan, or perhaps she has thrown around some numbers about "uptake" relative to spots that lit up on your PET scan. There may have been talk of your prognosis. She has also given you "the look," a look you are likely going to have to get used to in the coming weeks. "The look" is one of sorrow, sometimes pity, and my sense is that it is also one of introspection—an outward and quite unintentional indication that the person talking to you has been reminded that she, too, is mortal. You also may have made the mistake of asking, "How long do I have?" and she—more than likely—compounded your innocent mistake by telling you what the latest general statistics on this topic are, all while assuming you know what to make of such statistics.

If you were with a loved one or friend for this meeting, you both likely walked out of this meeting in a state of shock. Much of what was said was intellectually confusing, but not the most important words. You will never forget *those* words. Life presents us with days that are never forgotten. This was one of those days. You have just been told that you are on the threshold of death. The meeting with your oncologist is over, and you have now crossed the threshold of your home, your personal Rubicon. You are settled into familiar surroundings, and whether you like it or not, you have an immediate decision to make: Are you going to accept the fate just described to you, or are you going to fight?

Put very succinctly, are you going to rebel and fight, or are you going to allow yourself to assume the more tempting role of becoming a victim?

The issue is just this simple. You may not seem to have the energy to fight. Perhaps you are quite tired. You obviously are not feeling well. Perhaps you are even in great pain. You also may sense that people are feeling sorry for you, and you do, in some sense, feel like a victim. Perhaps if you have been a smoker, you sense that you *deserve* this fate. Perhaps the financial implications of any such fight are daunting. And let's be brutally honest: perhaps, deep down inside, the idea of checking out doesn't seem all that bad. In the beginning, I certainly experienced some of these thoughts.

Why decide to fight when the odds are, theoretically, so seemingly against you? I cannot answer these specific questions for you.

I can, however, tell you my thought process after the meeting in January of 2020. After much contemplation, my thought process was this: I would fight, and I would rebel against this disease—if not for myself—at least for my wife and daughter. I had spent three decades doing nothing *but* fighting on behalf of clients, not accepting defeat, and leaving nothing to chance because of any lack of effort. I had missed many family weekends and evenings while in trial, preparing for trial, or traveling to hearings and depositions on behalf of clients. I had fought hard and fair my entire life as a trial lawyer.

I decided that I owed no less than that same effort to my wife and daughter, to my family, and to my friends. When I was first diagnosed, more than a few friends said the same thing to me, more or less: "If anybody can beat this, you can." I listened to these friends, but more importantly, in the context of the gathering of so much information and the absorbing of such shocking news, I listened to my inner voice and made a decision. I decided that I was built for such a fight and that I would survive. I sent my wife a text dated January 23, 2020, within seventy-two hours of my formal diagnosis. The text said the following: *I know this sounds very weird, but I believe I am already healed. Now it's just a matter of working out the paces.*

As you learned in the preface, my wife had occasion to remind me of this decision during the worst of that first bout of chemotherapy. You may need reminders too, even after a firm decision. Sometimes, this reminder will come from your inner voice.

"Radical Remission survivors believe it is vital to check with your intuition before taking any sort of healing plan. Interestingly, this belief goes against typical Western medicine thinking, which usually removes patients from the planning process while the expert doctors determine what is wrong with their bodies and how to fix it."[28] Prior to sending the text to Rebecca, my inner intuitive voice told me it was time to fight and to go all in for this fight. Listening to this voice was critical, even though I hadn't yet "worked out" the paces. "Nearly all survivors in nearly *every* survival setting report what they call 'the voice.' It tells them what to do. It is the speaking, rational side of the brain, the one that processes language, the wellspring of reason."[29] I listened to that inner voice. I specifically committed to crossing my personal Rubicon.

Some do not like the term "fight" in this context, and I understand this perspective. Martial metaphors, such as "the war on cancer," or one's "battle with cancer," are perhaps too common in the cancer world. But let's again be very blunt about this: your situation is very grave. This is not a time to get hung up on one's choice of metaphors.

In early 2020, when I was gathering books and other resources in my home office relative to the fight ahead, I joked with my wife that I was naming that office the "War Room." I had a four-foot-by-six-foot whiteboard hung on a wall with treatment options written out, supplements I needed to take, mental game exercises I planned to execute, doctors' appointments, further reading, and so on. Eventually, however, we changed the name of that room to the "Peace Room." Converting my office from a war room to a peace room was, thankfully, a luxury I was afforded over time. I lived long enough to surrender the idea of war and replace it with peace. This was no small thing, and I will discuss this transition in a later chapter.

But we are talking about Phase One here, the first ninety days. In those first ninety days, when you are sick, when you are in shock, and you are more than likely beginning treatments that make those outside the cancer world flinch, make no mistake: you are in a *fight* for your life. As my karate sensei likes to say, "Time to stop yakking and start smacking." Reject the prognosis. Fix your resolve. Discover, refine, and then summon your will to live.

Some form of surrender and acceptance will have its place later, as I will discuss below. For now, if you wish to survive stage IV lung cancer, you had better be or become a fighter. "You must remain obstinate and decide to survive."[30] You had better develop an edge to your game, so to speak.

o o o

The title of this chapter is "Crossing the Rubicon." Rubicon was the name of a river in Ancient Rome, crossed by Julius Caesar in 49 BC. Once Julius Caesar crossed the river Rubicon on his way back to Rome, he knew civil war would ensue, eventually leading to his becoming a dictator. Everything would change. Once he made this ultimate decision, a line had been crossed. "Crossing the Rubicon" means passing the point of no return. And according to legend, Caesar was heard to say, before crossing, "Alea iacta est" (The die is cast). I knew when I sent my wife the January 23 text that the die was cast. I trust you now see why this chapter is named as it is.

What does it mean to be a rebel or a fighter in this context? I will throw out a couple of ideas.

First, you must know your opponent. "Educating yourself about your particular form of cancer is one of the most important and empowering things you can do after you've received your diagnosis."[31] Second, you must learn to ask questions, to get outside of your comfort zone around authority figures—such as doctors—and to make your own judgments. Again, Gonzales perhaps puts it too strongly, where he says about cancer survivors that "the medical staff observes that they are 'bad patients,' unruly, troublesome. ... They question everything,"[32] but he is not far from a core truth.

Third, and this is especially true in Phase One, you must resist the temptation to become a victim. This will be a great temptation. People of goodwill are going to feel sorry for you even if they don't say so out loud. You cannot use this as permission to play the victim. Fighters are not victims. You truly have no time to play the victim. I am no mind reader, but every time I have entered a treatment waiting room for chemotherapy or radiation in the past five years, I have consciously looked at the room to make an assessment of the ratio of those with a victim's guise and those who are the fighters. The ratio sometimes tends to favor the victims, and the fighters are usually quite obvious.

Everybody in the room needs to be a fighter.

Not long after my diagnosis, I came across the already-quoted book written by Annette and Richard Bloch. Near the beginning of the book, Bloch succinctly states the issue for the newly diagnosed: "I am not trying to say that everyone can beat cancer. Certainly some people are going to die from it, no matter what they do. I am saying, however, that if a person does not try, there is no way they can beat it. If they do try, they have a chance... To me, there was nothing worse than waiting to die with no hope. Whatever treatments I went through did not compare to the lack of hope I had the first five days after diagnosis. *I was fighting to live rather than waiting to die.*"[33]

So, the question is this simple: Are you willing to cross *your* personal Rubicon? This is a conscious decision, and here, in Phase One, there is no time to waste. Becoming *your* best form of a fighter in this context will be your greatest act of love you can provide for your family and friends.

This act of love will also be what sustains you during the rough times ahead, during Phase One and beyond.

Chapter 3: *Becoming a Happy, Optimistic Warrior*

From the moment I was diagnosed, I knew it was going to be a challenge and a grim one at that. Yet at the same time, I felt it could also be viewed as a journey, an adventure that I was about to embark upon. Instead of hanging my head low and feeling sorry for myself, I decided to take as upbeat an approach as possible.

—MICHAEL LLOYD, *Beating Crazy Odds*

MAKING THE DECISION TO FIGHT DOES NOT MEAN DECIDING TO become an *angry* fighter.

Two or three months after being diagnosed, and just before starting chemotherapy, I was playing golf with a couple of my regular golfing buddies on a balmy spring day. Golfing was one of the few social outings available during the COVID pandemic. One of my best pals had sort of put one over on me that day. A new guy—his name was Freddie—was joining our golf group, and it just so happened that Freddie was, like my mentor Mark I mentioned earlier, a ten-year survivor of stage IV esophageal cancer. My pal Geno had orchestrated this encounter, I think, on purpose.

Freddie was a great guy and could hit the ball a mile, even with a lit cigarette hanging out of his mouth. Freddie was clearly a fighter. He was not someone you would think of as a "terminal" throat cancer survivor, and not just because of the cigarette hanging out of his mouth. Having not yet started chemotherapy, I marveled that this guy had been through chemotherapy and radiation many moons ago and had lived to talk about it. Just his presence inspired me.

At about the halfway point in the game, I asked Freddie how he had survived throat cancer and what his advice was for me, just beginning the worst of the upcoming treatments.

One thing about Freddie that I immediately appreciated: he did not give me "the look." Members of the club do not usually give each other the look, in my experience. In response to my question, however, he did look me straight in the eye and said, "You've gotta have a positive attitude. That's the key to this thing." And when he said, "this thing," he motioned and waved with his arm as if pointing to membership in the club. I had already been doing some research about cancer survivors, and I had seen the importance of attitude as a through-line. I nodded and said thanks. Then he stepped up and drove the ball about forty yards past me.

Very simple advice. You need to have a positive attitude. Such simple advice that it almost sounds absurd. But this simple advice is *not* absurd. Having a positive attitude is simple but not easy, especially in the middle of a fight. Freddie was telling me I needed to become a happy warrior. Later on, I would read Laurence Gonzalez's book and read this: "Survival is a simple test. There's only one right answer, but cheating is allowed."[34] What is the simplest way to cheat? "Positive Mental Attitude."[35]

"Positive Mental Attitude" has the faint whiff of bullshit, does it not? How can some New Age–sounding phrase help in surviving cancer? It helps more than you might guess. In some of the research I had done before and after that day on the golf course I described, I had run across an article written by the world-famous evolutionary biologist Stephen Jay Gould. I had heard of Gould before but wasn't aware that in the early 1980s while he was in his early forties, he had been diagnosed with peritoneal mesothelioma, a fairly rare cancer that, at the time, had a median survival rate of eight months. He lived twenty years past that diagnosis.

In Gould's article, after touching upon some of the statistical traps inherent in looking at survival rates, Gould struck at the heart of the matter: "Attitude clearly matters in fighting cancer. We don't know why. ... But match people with the same cancer for age, class, health, and socio-economic status, and, in general, those with positive attitudes, with a strong purpose and will for living, with commitment to struggle, and with an active response to aiding their own treatment and not just a passive acceptance of anything doctors say tend to live longer."[36]

There you have it, in a nutshell, from a world-class scientist. Attitude clearly matters. Attitude manifests in one's response to treatments, one's response to what the doctors might say, and it also bears on one's will for living.

I agree with Bloch, Gonzales, Gould, and Freddie. I don't know *why* attitude matters, but I do know that it does. Gould's road map for obtaining such an attitude could not have rung truer: have a strong will and purpose for living; have a commitment to the struggle; have an active response to aiding your own treatment; do not passively accept the judgments of doctors.

These are some of the constituent parts of having a good attitude.

But Gould's additional comments in the article resonate as well: "A few months [after my diagnosis] I asked Sir Peter Medawar, my personal scientific guru and a Nobelist in immunology, what the best prescription for success against cancer might be. 'A sanguine personality,' he replied."[37]

Cancer is, at bottom, the result of a failure of the immune system. Here, a Nobelist in immunology and a guru to one of the world's foremost scientists is saying the *best* prescription against cancer is a sanguine personality, defined in Webster's Dictionary as "marked by eager hopefulness; confidently optimistic." Gould then ended his essay with beautiful language, alluding to the famous Dylan Thomas poem, language that anybody in Phase One would do well to hold near and dear: "For most situations ... I prefer the more martial view that death is the ultimate enemy—and I find nothing reproachable in those who rage against the dying of the light."[38]

There you have it. You are indeed in the fight of your life. But raging against the dying of the light does not mean to do so with *rage*. Why not become a happy warrior in that fight? Doing so might just save your life.

Chapter 4: *Getting a Second Opinion*

Many cancer patients are dying, not because treatments are not available, but because the initial physician failed to offer the best possible treatment.

—Richard and Annette Bloch Family Foundation website

YOU MAY FIND IT ODD THAT WE ARE WELL INTO PART I, WHICH focuses on Phase One, and I still haven't specifically discussed any recommended cancer treatments. The reason I have not discussed cancer treatments is, quite simply, that I am not an oncologist, and I know nothing about your pathology. Thankfully, there seem to be many oncologists out there, so why accept the opinion of the first one you meet?

I am not trying to be cute here. Your cancer treatments are a subject to be determined by you and your trusted medical advisers. In my case, my trusted medical advisers disagreed on the course of medical treatments after my diagnosis. My local oncologist suggested a cutting-edge course of treatment that involved immunotherapy, something I had only ever heard about because of the nonstop television advertisements by drug companies during my golf and football watching. In contrast, my national oncologist—truly one of the most impressively capable persons I have ever met—suggested a much simpler standard treatment. She suggested that I have my lung tumor radiated for three weeks and then undergo six cycles of platinum-based chemotherapy. After that, she recommended that we reassess whether maintenance chemotherapy was appropriate after the standard regimen was finished. In addition, I met with a nationally recognized integrative oncologist, who gave me advice about the looming options on the table and also recommended parallel treatments that would work in tandem with traditional treatment options.

The actual decision among these options was mine, and the tipping point was strategic: the second opinion in favor of the standard treatment option would allow me to hold back on the immunotherapy option for a later date if it ever were needed. In other words, the standard radiation/chemotherapy option maintained the possibility of future immunotherapy, but the converse of this was *not* necessarily true. My understanding was that if I took the immunotherapy option first, there might be no second bite at that apple.

"Many cancer patients are dying, not because treatments are not available, but because the physician failed to offer the best possible treatment."[39] With all of this in mind, I decided to go with standard radiation and then chemotherapy. No razzle-dazzle moves. No cutting-edge therapies. No clinical trials either. This, I think, has turned out to be the right path, but I was by no means certain of this in real time.

You are undoubtedly going to have to go through some version of this process in Phase One. The most *comfortable* course would be to accept the first opinion you receive about treatments. But surviving advanced cancer of any kind does not provide many *comfortable* options. I hope you have the option of obtaining, as I did, a second opinion on your course of treatment. I also hope you have the option of obtaining, as I did, an additional opinion from an integrative oncologist. Integrative oncologists combine, in my opinion, the best of both worlds—medical expertise in traditional cancer treatments with an open mind about alternative treatments available to the confused and fearful cancer patient.

Obviously, every person's situation is different—financially, psychologically, and perhaps equally important here, geographically. A person with stage IV NSCLC who lives in the middle of North Dakota does not have the same readily available options as a person with the same diagnosis who lives in Houston, Texas, probably the oncology capital of the world. Here, however, you must leave no stone unturned. You must be bold. You must be willing to rebel in the sense of leaving no stone unturned, even if this runs the risk of getting outside your comfort zone or offending your initial oncologist.

There are many different ways to expend your limited energy in Phase One, but in my opinion, the most important *treatment* action you can take in Phase One is to obtain a second opinion from a traditional oncologist and then, ideally, a *third* opinion from an integrative oncologist. This problem, ironically, may be one of the only medical "favors" the COVID pandemic has given the cancer patient: telehealth second and third opinions are now an option for the geographically, logistically, and even financially challenged.

Fortune favors the bold. You cannot accept discussions about how long you have to live. You are a happy warrior who has committed to cross the Rubicon. The war has not yet truly started, but it is coming. Now is the time for rebellious hope. Do not accept the first piece of advice you have been given. Get a second opinion about your treatment options. Ideally, get a third one too.

Chapter 5: *Confronting the "Why" Question*

There is a common refrain among cancer patients: why me? My response is, why not me?

—MICHAEL WEITZ, MD

THERE IS AN IMPORTANT ISSUE THAT CANNOT HELP BUT PRESENT itself at some point in Phase One, not only for NSCLC patients but also for any kind of cancer patient. Here, for lack of another way of putting it, I am going to suggest that—consciously or unconsciously—you are likely going to have to confront the "meaning" of your getting what is considered a terminal form of cancer.

This issue of meaning is sometimes broached by unfortunate remarks of well-meaning others. You have been diagnosed with lung cancer. Lung cancer seems to be one of the few types of cancer that still carries with it the tinge of personal culpability. I cannot tell you how many times I was asked after my diagnosis some version of the following questions: "How did you get lung cancer?" or, "You are not a smoker, are you?" or, "What was your diet like?"

Are people with pancreatic cancer asked these questions? Maybe, but I have my doubts. At first, I tried to actually *answer* these questions, which led to some fairly frustrating discussions. After a time, I realized that, fundamentally, these were not questions at all in the classic sense. The person asking the question was not really seeking *information* but was quite unconsciously and inadvertently stating out loud their fear that they, too, might someday be in my shoes. They were hoping, without even knowing it, that I somehow "caught" cancer because of my actions, actions that might make them feel better about avoiding the disease.

The questions and comments of others, at least for me, could fairly readily be dismissed. I am not going to claim I modeled Mother Teresa in each and every one of these conversations. I found them fairly annoying, and depending upon the seeming good faith of the "question," I answered more or less forthrightly. When especially annoyed by the topic, I would sometimes bring up the fact that a good friend I had met during my cancer treatments had an eight-month-old baby going through chemotherapy and that, as far as I could tell, that baby was not a smoker and had done nothing in her life to "deserve" being diagnosed with cancer. This example would bring such conversations to a screeching halt. When in a more compassionate mood, I realized that these questions, and even "the look," were really examples of others trying to figure out the meaning of cancer.

The question is going to present itself whether you like it or not: Is there a meaning to your cancer? Here, you must rebel against any attempted meanings attributed to your cancer imposed upon you—expressly or otherwise—by others.

What do I mean by this?

o   o   o

Ken Wilber is a prolific intellectual, philosopher, and writer. He has written at least fifty books, primarily concerned with consciousness, personal transformation, and even *A Theory of Everything*.[40] Wilber thinks deeply about any issue that comes across the screen of his consciousness.

In the mid-1980s, Wilber married the love of his life, Terry Killam. Within a week of their marriage, Terry was diagnosed with stage II breast cancer. Roughly five years later, after several surgeries, radiation, brutal chemotherapy, and a great deal of then-cutting-edge alternative cancer treatments, Treya (during these treatments, she changed her first name from Terry to Treya) died of cancer. Treya fought the good fight as a happy warrior and with boldness. Treya was and is one of the notorious ones.

The story of Ken and Treya's marriage and battle with cancer can be found in Ken Wilber's book, *Grace and Grit*, written in 1991.[41] I highly recommend this uncompromisingly honest memoir of marriage and cancer. Reading the book in my third year of survival, having survived two separate cancers, I was taken aback to see how much *each* cancer story shares commonality with other cancer stories. But the twist with Wilber's book is his capacious mind and comfort in addressing the big picture issues broached by a cancer diagnosis.

The most penetrating of Wilber's insights involves the question of meaning and, specifically, the responsibility for finding meaning in the context of cancer. Because of its power, I am going to quote Wilber's insights extensively: "In any disease, a person is confronted with two very different entities. One, the person with the actual disease process itself—a broken bone, a case of influenza, a heart attack, a malignant tumor. Call this aspect of disease 'illness.' Cancer, for example, is an illness, a specific disease with medical and scientific dimensions. Illness is more or less value-free; it's not true or false, good or bad, it just is—just like a mountain isn't good or bad, it just is."[42]

So far, so good. The smear on your CT scan is representative of an object within your torso. There is no inherent meaning to that smear or the object it represents.

This first distinction described by Wilber was especially resonant with me when I was diagnosed with prostate cancer. I distinctly recall telling my lung oncologist, after the diagnosis from the urology oncologist, those precise words: "Prostate cancer is just a thing. That's all." This thoughtful, compassionate doctor let out a rare laugh in response to my cockiness. I then added, "I scoff at prostate cancer." A rather more muted and uncomfortable laugh then ensued. But I meant it. I didn't realize it at the time, but I was unconsciously *living* the point made by Wilber, whose book I hadn't yet read. Unlike lung cancer, nobody really thinks a prostate cancer patient is *responsible* for his condition.

In other words, I *instinctively* attached *zero* meaning to having the illness known as prostate cancer. Wilber's second distinction captures what I instinctively understood. Here is how he explains it:

> But two, the person is also faced with how his or her society or culture deals with that illness—with all the judgments, fears, hopes, myths, stories, values, and meanings that a particular society hangs on each illness. Call this aspect of disease "sickness". Cancer is not only an illness, a scientific and medical phenomenon; it is also a sickness, a phenomenon loaded with cultural and social meanings. Science tells you when and how you are ill; your particular culture or subculture tells when and how you are sick.[43]

The key distinction is between illness and sickness.

Why is this distinction so important? "It is not enough to know *that* I have a disease; *that* I have a disease is my illness. But I also need to know *why* I have that disease. Why me? What does it mean? What did I do wrong? How did this happen? I need, in other words, to attach some sort of *meaning* to this illness."[44] Wilber—who seemingly can't help but draw out unexpected philosophical conclusions in every paragraph of his writings—then wraps up his point: "Men and women are condemned to meaning, condemned to values and judgments." Why does this matter? "Thus, it is through science that I seek to explain my illness ... but it is through my society that I seek to *understand* my sickness—what does it mean?"[45] Wilber concludes, "And the point is that the meaning of that sickness—negative or positive, redemptive or punitive, supportive or condemnatory—can have an enormous impact on me and the course of my disease; *the sickness is often more destructive than the illness*"[46] (emphasis added).

This latter point is worth repeating: the sickness is often more destructive than the illness. And, I suspect, this distinction between an illness and a sickness is especially important for those with lung cancer.

The newly diagnosed stage IV lung cancer patient will be tempted to impose value judgments on his or her illness. This will be especially tempting for smokers and former smokers, but I can attest that this temptation exists for never-smokers as well. I cannot tell you how to attribute meaning after a diagnosis, whether you are in the midst of Phase One or have the (relative) luxury afforded in later phases of survival outlined in this book. Again, I cannot tell you *what* meaning to attach to your illness, but I can offer the reminder that it is *you* who is responsible for attributing meaning—if any—to your sickness. Not society. Not inquisitive and well-meaning friends. Not even your doctor, your pastor, or your spiritual adviser. Not your family members. Not gauzy television commercials. Not Ken Wilber or me.

o o o

In case you might find it interesting, I can tell you what meaning I have attached to my illness, the diagnosis of advanced lung cancer. The answer is quite simple, if disappointing: I have attached zero meaning to the illness. My having lung cancer *is*. Just like my having had prostate cancer. My lung cancer simply *is what it is*. To repeat a quote at the beginning of this section, "People get cancer, and I am one of the people."[47]

"Science" cannot tell me what caused either of the cancers found in my body, just like science cannot tell me why my friend's eight-month-old daughter is going through chemotherapy or why a friend of a friend was just recently diagnosed with ALS. Things happen. Bad things happen. We have far less control over these things than anybody would like to contemplate or admit. To use Wilber's terms, I have, in effect, sidestepped the question of meaning, and I do not consider my cancer to be a sickness. Lung cancer is simply an illness, and your rebellious hope should be to render it a *chronic* illness, just like that person in your family or circle of friends with multiple sclerosis, diabetes, or many other types of lifelong conditions.

It is up to *you* to find meaning or nonmeaning for your illness. But you should do so consciously, not through societal osmosis or default.

Chapter 6: *Confronting the Prospect of Death*

When Samurai Warriors went into battle, they carried a little purse containing the money for their funeral and everything that was necessary. If you go into battle fearlessly accepting the possibility of death and almost embracing it, you have a much better chance of fighting well, and in fact winning, than if you go into battle scared to death.

—Rick Fields, quoted by Ernest H. Rosenbaum and
Isadora H. Rosenbaum, *Inner Fire*, 93

Given the survival rates applicable to Phase One, there is a topic that may well be regarded as *the* topic to address in Phase One.

The topic is your potential death.

One's willingness and ability to confront one's death, in my experience, has a direct effect on survival, and there is a growing body of research "showing that facing death better helps people live longer with cancer."[48] Put another way, "fear keeps the body stuck in fight or flight mode, which means that the body cannot switch to rest-and-repair mode."[49]

I have gone back and forth about whether and how to write this particular chapter. I am as reluctant to discuss death as anybody else in our Western culture, a culture that has nearly extinguished any reasoned or rational discussion of death or at least sanitized the topic beyond recognition. It would be rather presumptuous of me to think there was something original to say on this important subject. But even from a simple perspective of *enhancing survival*, the topic cannot be avoided.

First, let me tell you a true story. In my early fifties, I undertook a fairly comprehensive study of Stoicism, the philosophical doctrine that dominated the Greek and Roman societies of the ancient world. You may know that Stoicism has made something of a comeback in early twenty-first-century American culture. My focus during this Stoicism phase was on the Roman Stoics, especially Marcus Aurelius, the great emperor of Rome in the second century, who, in his spare time during the evenings, while also fighting the barbarian hordes thousands of miles from his home, wrote his famous *Meditations*. In the *Meditations*, Marcus contemplated the approach of his own death. As a practicing Stoic, Marcus outlined how he practiced the Stoic doctrine called *memento mori*. *Momento mori* means, more or less, "remember that you have to die."[50]

In my study of the *Meditations*, I was moved by Marcus's willingness to confront death. I was moved that he did not look the other way. In fact, I carried a medallion in my pocket, which I still have, with the phrase *Memento Mori* on it. On one side of the medallion is a skull and an hourglass. On the other side is the phrase "You could leave life right now." The concept of *memento mori* was of great significance to me. I considered its contemplation one of the key spiritual practices in my life in the first half of my fifties. But—and this is important—I was a healthy man. Then, as you know, a well-meaning oncologist told me that, without effective treatment, I had only a few months to live.

Marcus Aurelius had taught me the theory and a notion of the practice of an important spiritual principle. *Cancer taught me the lived experience memento mori.* This is the difference between reading a menu and tasting the food. I do not carry the medallion in my pocket anymore. There is no need to do that. I now know what *memento mori* actually means. In this respect, cancer has been one of my life's greatest blessings. I know any description of cancer as a blessing sounds extremely weird, but I can assure you this has been true for me.

o o o

Cancer—stage IV lung cancer—has given you an opportunity to figure out what really matters and to make friends with death. If you do not address this subject, so to speak, consciously, you are more than likely going to do so subconsciously. *Every* survivor must confront this issue. This issue is inherent in survival itself, whether you are Marcus Aurelius fighting the barbarians or about to undertake yet another chemotherapy treatment: "'Fortitude is necessary, and patience and courtesy and modesty and decorum, and a will, in what may for the *moment* seem to be the worst of worlds, to *do* one's best.' ... The same applies to any survival situation."[51]

It is a radical, rebellious act in today's culture to look death in the eye, but most importantly for our purposes, doing so actually enhances the opportunity for long-term survival. "Many Radical Remission survivors have taken some time to look death in the face and accept its inevitability. However, they also realize that no one—not even their doctors—can know for sure when they are going to die."[52] Those who die instant deaths, those in car crashes, or who suffer heart attacks are not given this blessing. The child with cancer is not really given this blessing, as she likely has no tools to process such a blessing.

Which leads to, perhaps, my most important advice to you in Phase One: rebel against the notion that cancer is your curse and accept it as a blessing instead. You were *eventually* going to need to confront the approach of your certain death. That day just came much sooner than you thought it might. Accept the blessing cancer has provided you—use it as an opportunity to experience *memento mori*.

Do yourself a favor and look death in the eye. Do not run from death. Instead, flip the script. Look at the crisis confronting you as a blessing.

This is what deep survivors do.

Chapter 7: *Employing the Mental Game of Visualization*

The mind is a powerful healing tool. Imagery (visualization) has harnessed the power of mind through various therapies for centuries. ... The more specific the visualization, the more helpful it will likely be.
        —JOHNS HOPKINS MEDICINE, *What Is Imagery?*

THE LIKELIHOOD OF BEING OVERWHELMED DURING PHASE ONE cannot be underestimated.

Your life has been upended. You are drinking out of informational and psychological fire hoses. You are meeting with doctors to whom it is very tempting to delegate life-or-death decisions. You may even need to get "your affairs in order." All of these arrows are coming straight at you while you feel terrible, are working out how you are going to remain employed, and, most importantly, while your loved ones are also in distress and despair.

You are seeking second and maybe third opinions, and you are girding for what is quite literally the fight of your life.

In the context of all of this, it may seem absurd that I suggest that you add something else to your plate, let alone a mental exercise that is called "visualization." I promise you this is not some New Age trick for the weak-minded. World-class experts in any number of fields undertake this strategy *all the time*. I also promise you that this is a strategy I employed and that, yes, you have time to do this, even and especially in Phase One. This

mental exercise will take you about thirty to sixty minutes to prepare as an initial matter, and then it will take you no more than
five minutes or so to execute on a regular basis.

What is visualization? Specifically, what is the type of visualization I am suggesting?

Bear with me because I am about to talk about golf again.
Everybody has heard of Jack Nicklaus, one of the greatest golfers
of all time. Many are aware that he has won more major cham-
pionships than any other golfer. How did he do this? What does
Jack Nicklaus claim to have been his secret to success? Nicklaus
"went to the movies." Listen to how Jack Nicklaus describes this:
"Many years ago I wrote, 'I never hit a shot, even in practice, without having a very sharp, in-focus picture of it in my head. It's like
a color movie.' I still feel that way today. You visualize what you're
trying to do, then you figure what swing will fit ... your shot, then
you put all the pieces together to play it. Of course, I don't say all
that to myself. I just do it. It happens naturally."[53] If you would
like to see a modern golfer implement Nicklaus's advice, I suggest you watch (or google a video of) the pro golfer Jason Day.
Before each shot, you can see Day stand behind the ball, his eyes
partially shut and fluttering just a bit. Day is engaged in what
is called "outcome visualization." That is one reason why he was
once the number one player in the world.

As a trial lawyer for over three decades, I had used visualization techniques for at least twenty years. For instance, I rarely, if
ever, verbally rehearsed an opening statement or closing argu-
ment in any of the cases I have tried since 1987. Instead, I would
prepare a detailed, written outline of my presentation and then
sit and visualize myself making the presentation. That was how I
practiced my arguments. I always viewed my lack of conventional
practice or rehearsal to allow for a more authentic presentation.

Given this history, I was familiar with the concept of visualization after my diagnosis and was comfortable that this process had served me well over the years in the one professional area in which I possess some expertise.

I adjusted the visualizations required after my diagnosis to include outcome visualization, the mental technique of creating a picture in your mind of a specific outcome. In Phase One, for instance, one outcome visualization might be for you to imagine a meeting with your oncologist after ninety days to discuss and review a positive scan result. In that visualization, you would be as specific as possible in terms of imagining the treatment room, the look and demeanor of your doctor and nurse, and even the feeling of your butt on the patient chair. Then you might imagine your doctor telling you that (as was applicable in my case) the tumor in your right lung has shrunk and that any metastasis has halted.

When I was going through my treatments, I did not use the Phase-related timing paradigm we have been discussing in this book. I wasn't aware of such phases, as no study I was aware of had come out involving such phases. I did not think about Phase One, Phase Two, and so on. But I *did* visualize a very specific outcome of one of my first scans after those three weeks of radiation. I even visualized my oncologist's accent when delivering the news, with her understated but very pleasant demeanor.

Later in this book, I will further describe some additional outcome visualizations I used and am using. In total, during Phases One and Two, I visualized seven different outcomes, ranging from being present at Jacqulyn's graduation ceremony to a specific vacation with my family on Lake Michigan, at a beach house, where we all celebrated my having survived eighteen months after diagnosis. All but one of my outcome visualizations actually came true. The single outcome that didn't come to pass was, ironically, related to golf, but you've already heard enough about golf in a book about surviving cancer.

Outcome visualization is an example of what I have termed the "parallel silo" approach to cancer treatments. Spending two to three minutes visualizing a desired outcome in a relaxed state of mind and *emotionally believing* that the outcome will come to pass is itself a treatment that runs parallel to your other treatments. I think it is also important to consider visualizing events occurring apart from your specific cancer treatments, including any potential celebrations on your horizon. In other words, try to disperse your visualizations across a diverse range of potential future events.

It is in this context the comments that I allude to throughout this book are so relevant: cancer is far and away medical science's most mysterious disease. If this is true, let's not pretend that there is *only one way to be a cancer patient*. Let us also not pretend that we know things about how alternative treatments work against cancer when we most assuredly do not. And finally, let's not ignore the lessons of others, such as world-class athletes and business leaders who use such techniques to enhance or influence improbable outcomes.

To reiterate, you have at your disposal any number of parallel silos of treatment for your condition. You may or may not agree with the theoretical paradigms that drive those parallel silos, but this is no time for intellectual pride. In other words, please do not allow predetermined belief systems to impede a potential avenue of recovery. Your role as a hopeful rebel in Phase One and beyond is to engage as many parallel silos as possible *as long as no treatment silo diminishes the efficacy of your standard treatments*. Do not worry about theoretical paradigms right now. Take as inspiration the position of Sir Isaac Newton, the man who discovered gravity but admitted that he had no idea *why* gravity worked the way it did. His position was *"hypothesis non fingo"*—in other words, he "feigned no hypothesis" as to why it worked the way it did.

Visualization *of any kind* is a perfect example of this. I do not claim to know why or how visualization works, although I could hazard some decent guesses, which would be well beyond the scope of this book. Visualization in no way impairs your radiation, chemotherapy, surgery, or immunotherapy silos. In fact, it may do just the opposite. In a comparative study conducted in September–October 2010 and written up in the *Cancer Nursing* 33(5), the authors noted "statistically significant results" for those who used "relaxation with visualization."[54] Other studies have explored this connection as well.[55]

Tapping into various elements of the mental game of cancer is probably *the* core element of the "parallel silo" strategy for surviving stage IV lung cancer, and visualization can simply and easily become a component of that mental game. Visualization "is a very powerful technique ... and you can do it any way that you want."[56]

Pick one visualization that resonates for you and is applicable to Phase One. Be very specific. Commit to this visualization at least once per day. This will take you less than five minutes per day. Once you become comfortable with this, add one or two more such visualizations. In this context, momentum begets momentum. You may be rather surprised where this momentum takes you.

PART II

Responsible Hope: Surviving the First Year after Diagnosis

Radical Remission survivors approach healing from a different perspective, where taking control of your healing is not only considered good but is actually essential for the healing process.

—KELLY TURNER, *Radical Remission*

The best thing a patient can do to strengthen his will to live is to get involved as an active participant in combatting his or her disease.

—ERNEST AND ISADORA ROSENBAUM,
"The Will To Live," Stanford Medical

Chapter 8: *Understanding the Importance of Responsible Hope*

Survivors are able to transform thought into action. They are willing to take risks to save themselves. .... They are able to break down very large jobs into small, management tasks. They set attainable goals and develop short-term plans to reach them. They are meticulous about doing these tasks well. They deal with what is within their power from moment to moment, hour to hour, day to day. They leave the rest behind.
—LAURENCE GONZALES, *Deep Survival*

WE LEARNED DURING PHASE ONE THAT REBELLIOUS HOPE requires pushing against conventional wisdom about your diagnosis. We learned some ways to turn this notion into action. In Phase Two, the remaining nine months of the year after your initial diagnosis, something almost the opposite of this is required: instead of pushing against, the central focus becomes a "pulling in," and that pulling in is the taking of personal responsibility for your health.

Phase Two is driven by *responsible hope*. "Hope is one of the most vital factors to effectively cope with the loss, uncertainty, and pain caused by cancer."[57] *Responsible hope* is the type of hope that self-generates when one takes personal responsibility for one's healing. In the words of Kelly Turner above, this is "essential for the healing process."

The ninety days of Phase One are a whirlwind, but they should calm down a bit after you learn that your scans are improving and you are still in the game. The transition to Phase Two allows for some breathing space to make something more of a *psychological* transition. This transition is primarily the transition from being the recipient of bad news and cancer treatments to being the gatherer of information about your disease and the quarterback of your treatments. Phase Two is the opportunity to move from a reactive mode to a more proactive mode. As the quotes above demonstrate, this transition is a critical part of the healing process.

It is well known in oncology circles that patients who take responsibility for their healing have the opportunity for better outcomes. As the doctor quoted in the book by the Blochs makes clear, there is a category of patients who will "do anything to get well." But recall that there is also that category of "50 to 60 percent [who] are willing to get better so long as the doctor does the work, and the medicine doesn't taste too bad."[58] In my experience in meeting with others recently diagnosed with cancer, I would estimate that about half of those I meet are willing to take this additional step, and there are about half who are, as the doctor quoted above states, inclined to let the doctors do all the work.

As you enter Phase Two, you will not discard the rebellious spirit we have already discussed but instead will benefit from *transforming* that spirit and rechanneling it into doing "whatever it takes" to *keep* surviving.

But what does "whatever it takes" mean, in fact?

Before one can assess what doing whatever it takes entails, one must first assess where he or she stands at the end of Phase One. The core element of this assessment is a deep understanding of survival rates.

Chapter 9: *Learning How to Assess Survival Rates*

I suspect most people, without training in statistics, would [assess statements about survival rates] as 'I will probably be dead in eight months'—the very conclusion that must be avoided, both because this formulation is false and because attitude matters so much.

—STEPHEN JAY GOULD, "The Median Isn't the Message"

LET'S FIRST TAKE ANOTHER LOOK AT WHERE YOU STAND AFTER Phase One.

The first act of taking personal responsibility requires, in my opinion, a deep understanding of survival rates for those with your disease. This applies to anybody with a recent cancer diagnosis, but in this chapter, I am going to focus on stage IV NSCLC. Your particular disease, unless it is NSCLC, is not likely to track the survival rates we discuss below.

This advice may seem counterintuitive in light of my earlier advice in Part I that one must reject all discussion of prognosis. It turns out, however, that an understanding of survival rates for stage IV NSCLC—which is not the same as accepting as true any prognosis about *your* particular circumstances—is a cause for some very good news. *The good news is that the survival rates applicable to those who survive Phase One increase dramatically.* You will recall that the 2020 study breaks down the time frames after Phase One in terms of survival time frames. Thus, in the one thousand or so NSCLC patient pool of the 2020 study, 737 individuals survived into Phase Two—they survived past ninety days and then were tracked for, initially, the remaining nine months of their first year after diagnosis.

Of those 737 individuals, 47 patients refused chemotherapy, radiation, and other traditional treatments, thus leaving 690 patients who received traditional chemotherapy, radiation, or surgery, or some combination of these. In the words of the authors, the median survival of the 47 patients who refused traditional treatments was "significantly worse" than their counterparts. In general, authors describe those 70 percent receiving standard treatments as follows: "Of these latter 690 patients, 42% were females, 58% males, median age 63 (range 27–85), 1-, 2-, 5-, and 10-year survival rates were 74%, 49%, 16%, and 5%. In total, 16% were alive with disease (AWD) at the last follow up." None of the "patients surviving 10 years were disease free, which is not surprising as all had stage IV disease at the start of the study."[59]

For the purposes of Phase Two, a translation of the information above can be summarized as follows: For those 690 patients who survived Phase One *and* then undertook standard treatments, 74 percent survived through Phase Two, a full year after diagnosis. Put another way, the raw survival rates of Phase Two are about the same as the survival rates of Phase One, although it must be borne in mind that this similar survival rate applies to a time frame spread out over nine months. In terms of raw numbers, of the 690 patients who survived Phase One, about 517 individuals went on to live at least a year. Or, to wrap up the numbers from the *beginning* of the study, after one year, there was about a 51.7 percent survival rate among the initial stage IV NSCLC population.

Returning to those who survive Phase One, of the 690 individuals who are treated with standard treatments, approximately half survived *two* years after diagnosis, that is, 345 individuals. Thus, in the original sample size of roughly one thousand NSCLC patients, roughly 34.5 percent survived two years. The survival rate of the sample of 690 who survived five years after their diagnosis was 16 percent (110 individuals), thus indicating a five-year survival rate from the roughly thousand-patient population of 11 percent. And finally, the survival rate of 5 percent ten years after diagnosis, when applied to the 690 who survived past the first three months is, when applied to the original sample of one thousand stage IV NSCLC patients, roughly 3.5 percent (35 individuals). The 2020 NSCLC Study indicates 35 or so of the original one thousand patients will be alive—albeit AWD—after ten years.

If one looks closely at these numbers, a remarkable trend begins to take shape. The trend is essentially this: assuming the stage IV NSCLC patient survives the first ninety days after diagnosis, statistically speaking, *at least 70 percent of all such survivors survived into the subsequent Phases.* This trend holds remarkably true through individual years one through five after diagnosis and is broken down in table 1 as follows:

Table 1

Survival rate after 3 months:	69% (691 individuals)
Survival rate after 12 months:	75% (517 individuals)
Survival rate after 24 months:	67% (345 individuals)
Survival rate after 36 months:	69% (238 individuals)
Survival rate after 48 months:	68% (161 individuals)
Survival rate after 60 months:	69% (111 individuals)

The authors of the 2020 NSCLC Study do not specifically break down the individual years after the five-year mark, but it turns out that the 70 percent survival rate holds firm, even after years one through five. *After* the five-year mark of the study, survival rates seem to increase to roughly 80 percent in subsequent years. To illustrate how my assumption about these remaining numbers comports with the 2020 Study, I have broken down some hypothetical survival rates for years six through ten in table 2 as follows:

Table 2

Survival rate after 72 months:	80% (88 individuals)
Survival rate after 84 months:	80% (71 individuals)
Survival rate after 96 months:	80% (56 individuals)
Survival rate after 108 months:	80% (45 individuals)
Survival rate after 120 months:	80% (36 individuals)

Again, table 2 above involves some assumptions not specifically elaborated in the 2020 study. In the table 2 breakdown of years six through ten, and in light of the actual number of survivors after ten years as addressed in the 2020 study, I have somewhat arbitrarily assumed a consistent survival rate across those years of 80 percent.

Again, the authors of the 2020 NSCLC Study did not really break years six through ten down individually, but given the relative consistency of the survival rates for years one through five, it is not too much of a leap to assume that a consistent survival rate of 80 percent, a rate that squares quite nicely with the endpoint data of the study (i.e., that 35 of the approximately one thousand persons diagnosed were still AWD). The uptick in survival rates after year five is also consistent with the rule of thumb in the cancer world that those who survive five years after diagnosis are at least somewhat more likely to survive for the long haul.

What the data from 2020 NSCLC Study demonstrates is a remarkably simple but powerful conclusion: statistically speaking, assuming one survives ninety days after diagnosis, approximately 70–80 percent of those diagnosed are likely to survive into each subsequent phase along the path of advanced NSCLC survival.

Do you now see why long-term cancer survivors, and especially those with advanced-stage NSCLC, are considered notorious?

o o o

This information is important as background information, but again, you—the person reading this book right now—are *not* a statistic. The failure to understand and contextualize statistics is the fundamental risk that exists in cancer survival. What do I mean by calling this a risk?

The risk is that a prognosis, or any literal reliance on the outcomes described in the 2020 NSCLC Study, can become a self-fulfilling prophecy. You've likely heard of the placebo effect: take a sugar pill and your mind "believes" it will have a healing effect. But the converse is true as well. "Placebo and nocebo pervade the whole history of medicine."[60] A common case of a nocebo is the "hex" put on another by somebody in authority, the classic example of this being a witch doctor. The nocebo effect kicks in when the person *believes* the hex, and the effects are just as real as with placebo. Yes, it makes sense to know the actual statistical information relevant to your disease, but it does *not* make sense to fail to put that statistical information in its proper perspective.

At this juncture, it makes sense to revisit Stephen Jay Gould, whom we met as an example of the happy warrior previously. The title of Gould's famous essay is important to remember: *The Median Isn't the Message*. We have already discussed Gould's discussion of the importance of a sanguine attitude, but the underlying purpose of that essay was to explain the potential traps of statistics to the newly diagnosed in the context of Gould's personal experience with stage IV cancer.

The first statistical distinction Gould describes is the difference between the mean and the median. "The mean represents our usual concept of an overall average—add up the items and divide them by the number of sharers (100 candy bars collected for five kids next Halloween will yield twenty for each in a fair world). The median, a different measure of central tendency, is the halfway point. If I line up five kids by height, the median is shorter than two and taller than the other two (who might have trouble getting their mean share of the candy)."[61]

Gould then applies this distinction to the prevalence of prognoses so common in the world of oncology. "The problem may be briefly stated: What does 'median mortality of eight months' signify in our vernacular? I suspect most people, without training in statistics, would read such a statement as, 'I will probably be dead in eight months,'—*the very conclusion that must be avoided, both because this formulation is false, and because attitude matters so much*."[62] Means and medians are abstractions. Gould then describes why this matters so much: "Therefore, I looked at the [survival rates involving] mesothelioma statistics quite differently—*and not only because I am an optimist who tends to see the doughnut instead of the hole, but primarily because I know that variation is itself the reality. I had to place myself amidst the variation*."[63]

Cancer survival can thus be viewed as a conscious strategy to place oneself "amidst the variation" of possible outcomes. In other words, to maximize the chances of landing on that side of the statistical variation in which one *becomes* a long-term survivor.

I hope I have incentivized you to google Gould's publicly available article and study it closely. You *must not accept* statistical survival rates at face value, but, at the same time, you must know where you stand. I have used the 2020 NSCLC Study as a handy basis to structure the time frames relevant to a stage IV NSCLC patient, but absent the context relevant to *you and your life*, the survival rates discussed in the study *are just that.*

In other words, the median is *not* the message.

o o o

Assuming your diagnosis is advanced NSCLC, perhaps your oncologist has already broken down these survival rates for you in connection with her discussion of your prognosis or in connection with the 2020 NSCLC Study. I hope she has, and I hope this chapter is redundant to discussions you have already had with your oncologist.

Assuming this has *not* been discussed, I hope you now see the good news inherent in your having survived into Phase Two, because the survival rates for Phase Two are markedly better than Phase One, and you now have great cause for optimism about becoming a long-term NSCLC survivor: you now have specific survival rate data to confirm why and how you can become an even happier warrior!

Let's now discuss how you can attack Phase Two and become one of the estimated 70 percent who make it to the second year and beyond. This begins by becoming a self-doctor and citizen-scientist, an important step that sets the stage for taking additional personal responsibility for your healing in Phase Two and beyond.

Chapter 10: *Becoming a Self-Doctor and "Citizen-Scientist"*

Shortly after I was diagnosed with terminal cancer in 1991, my personal n of 1 experiment began; its outcomes have been closely chronicled for a quarter of a century.

—GLENN SABIN, *n of 1*

MY MOTHER-IN-LAW, JACKIE BOGGS, WAS THE EPITOME OF A happy warrior. Before she died in 2013, she had spent over forty years living with multiple sclerosis. Rebecca and I were privileged to live near her parents for roughly twenty years, and we saw her mother battle multiple sclerosis valiantly as she made life adjustments, coordinated extensive medical treatments, rode the roller coaster of a life with MS, and responded to the long-term challenges of anybody who must deal with a chronic disease. One of Jackie's favorite comments about how she approached MS was that "you have to become your own best doctor." She did not read this in a book. This wisdom was the result of hard-won experience.

In early 2020, as I was studying the writings of Kelly Turner about radical remission very closely, I came across a cryptic yet very interesting description of one of the cancer survivors profiled in her book: "This began John's personal science experiment to save his life."[64] My ears perked up as I read that line, and I was reminded of Jackie's comments from the previous twenty-plus years. In reading Kelly Turner's comment, I realized that there was a truth in the notion of there being a *personal* path to cancer survival. Nothing shy of a "personal science experiment" was necessary.

○ ○ ○

You are, at some point, also going to have to conduct a personal science experiment on yourself if you are serious about surviving advanced lung cancer. What does this mean? Let's move away from the cancer world for a moment—a world fraught with mystery, pseudo-sciences, and claims for miracle cures—to a parallel world that seems to put cancer to shame in this regard, i.e., the world of Lyme disease.

In 2021, *New York Times* columnist Ross Douthat wrote a book about his experience with Lyme disease titled *The Deep Places: A Memoir of Illness and Discovery*.[65] I highly recommend his memoir to anybody reading this book, as it is a compelling tale for the survival of *any* disease, chronic or otherwise. The book demonstrates how, in the extreme and uncharted waters of dealing with Lyme disease, one must become an expert at self-doctoring while also managing to extract the best that traditional treatments have to offer. In *Deep Places*, Douthat emphasizes that each person faced with a serious disease is "an 'n' of only 1."[66] What Douthat means by an "n of 1" is that we all must, at some point, recognize that our particular disease as presented in our particular bodies is *sui generis*—of its own kind. As such, we must learn to "self-doctor" in the context of that illness or disease. Yes, there are usually, but not always, "standard" treatments available to those facing the challenge of cancer survival. But each person is different, and each person's *situation* is different. Each person's energy and resources are different. You must be willing to at least entertain the notion that *your* story of cancer survival is not written in the standard textbook authorized by Western medicine or in any current standard of care.

I have already alluded to the approach I have termed the "parallel silos" approach to cancer treatments. This means, essentially, a strategy of pursuing as many parallel or *complementary* treatments as possible in service of surviving cancer. Just as Douthat learned and as cancer survivor Glenn Sabin states in his book *n of 1*, some of these treatments will seem to work, and some will not. And here, if you will forgive me, a couple of dead horses deserve at last one more beating: "science" does not truly understand cancer even though it is certainly doing the best that it can for the present day; you are responsible for determining your healing; and finally, your course of treatment may not be the same as that cousin of the good friend who just told you yet another cancer anecdote.

No two cancers are alike. No two NSCLC cancers are alike, and certainly no two stage IV NSCLC cancers are alike either. And you are not like any other cancer survivor. This should be your operating assumption. My particular form of metastasis is not likely to be the same as yours. Our pathology may generally be similar, but our respective conditions are likely quite different. Your situation is unique. My pain tolerance is not likely the same as your pain tolerance. This distinction applies to many different conditions, and this recognition, the recognition that your condition is *unique*, should determine which particular treatment silos you pursue.

Deep cancer survival requires that you become a researcher "working on a study with a sample size, an "N" of only 1."[67] You and I are in the midst of a medical experiment in which the sample size for that experiment is one single person—ourselves. Glenn Sabin describes the mentality required: "I was now a citizen scientist. Amateur yes, I know. ... But I was determined not to be amateurish. I was absolutely serious about my research. I was conducting a study with an n of 1, the most precious single sample, myself."[68]

o o o

As you read further in this book, you will see some of the ways in which I conducted my own experiments, my own self-doctoring, and my own role as a citizen-scientist. You have already learned of one such experiment—my experiment and experience with visualization. You have also learned how my independent research into hyperbaric oxygen treatments led to additional treatments—covered by insurance, no less—that helped me recover from my first chemotherapy regimen. As we march further through part II, you will learn, for instance, how I utilized acupuncture and high-dose vitamins to, at a minimum, help me survive the effects of radiation and chemotherapy. You will also learn more about the paths taken by other long-term survivors.

My concern here is not with *how* you undertake these roles or *which* strategies you pursue. I am far more concerned *that* you consciously undertake these roles, as they are, in my opinion, the core elements of taking personal responsibility for your healing. Nobody can do this *for* you.

Chapter 11: *Learning to Communicate with Doctors*

Contemporary medicine prides itself on patient-centered care but it is startlingly inattentive—even actively indifferent—to patients' emotional needs. For patients with chronic illness, with its upheaval of life, this indifference poses a particular challenge. In chronic illness, the patient does not have a problem that can be solved quickly, but a disease to be managed, physically and psychologically. Such illnesses can be intractable, messy, mysterious. And doctors don't like to manage; they like to fix.

—MEGHAN O'ROURKE, *The Invisible Kingdom*

IN THE MIDST OF PHASE TWO, YOU ARE LIKELY RIGHT IN THE middle of treatments, feeling the effects of those treatments, and also, I hope, starting to get back on your feet.

You have probably already developed at least a medium-term relationship with your oncologist(s). You have also likely become something of a citizen-scientist about your condition, conducting a daily study with a sample size of 1. You certainly know a lot more today than you knew when you were diagnosed many months ago, but you are not a trained oncologist. This can present challenges, as more "problems and difficulties arise from poor communication than from anything else in all medical and nursing practice."[69]

This chapter discusses some of the challenges in communicating with oncologists. Some of what I say below is anecdotal, and it is pretty generalized. My goal with this chapter is to help you engage in *optimal* communication with your oncologist, and to do that, I think it important that you consider how most oncologists *think* and how they have been trained to *think*. The way oncologists *think* determines, in my opinion, a large part of how they *communicate*. I do not claim to be an expert on this, but in the past five years, I have been given medical advice or treatments from more than a dozen oncologists spanning the states of Kansas, Missouri, Minnesota, Texas, Tennessee, and Oregon. I have also cross-examined medical experts in at least a dozen different legal settings in the course of my law practice, and I have discussed this issue with dozens of other cancer survivors.

o o o

Let's start with the most obvious point. Oncologists, as a group, seem to have a wide range of bedside manners. You cannot allow yourself to be intimidated by any of these variations of bedside manners. Yes, I know—this is easier said than done.

In my career, I have appeared in front of some very intimidating judges. None of them hold a candle to the world-class oncologist from MD Anderson that I have told you about already. She was perfectly pleasant to me (and my law partner Mike—who accompanied me to our initial meeting as my scrivener), but Mike made the mistake of quite earnestly asking her, after about a half an hour of discussion, "Are you sure Paul has cancer?" or words to that effect. The look she gave my partner—one of my best friends, my karate sensei, and one of the best trial lawyers I know—was really one of the most comical episodes of these first sixty days after my diagnosis. She didn't *exactly* call him a dumbass asking dumbass questions, but she might as well have. No pun intended, but I had never seen Mike quite so quiescent.

Each of the oncologists I have mentioned above has had distinctly different communication styles. To illustrate, let me give you a couple of the statements that have been made to me by various oncologists since January 2020. You have already heard the details of my prognosis. You have also heard how I learned my condition was incurable. Absent proper context, those were certainly not pleasant conversations. On another occasion, after a very successful scan and a mutual decision (between my local oncologist, my wife, and me) that I could stop maintenance chemotherapy, I somewhat elatedly asked my oncologist, "What should I do next?"

I really had no idea what *to do* next now that I would be out of treatments, and we were both in just a little bit of shock. His response? "You might be thinking about what type of chemotherapy you might need next time." And thus did the balloon of that temporary elation pop. Afterward, Rebecca and I couldn't help but laugh.

Another example: when I was diagnosed with prostate cancer, I met with a local radiation oncologist to assess options among radiation, surgery, or "watching and waiting." This extremely competent and plainly quite pleasant young man hesitated as he was about to outline his recommendation about what I should do next. In the uncomfortable silence, I said, "Go ahead. There is nothing you can say that will offend me."

His response? "Well, there is a significant likelihood you are going to die of lung cancer, so I am not sure it really makes sense for you to treat the prostate cancer." It turned out I must have been bluffing: he actually *could* offend me. Because I wasn't sure I believed my ears, I read the clinical notes of our discussion the next day as they were posted to my medical chart. Yep, he did say what I thought he said.

Perhaps the most egregious example I have heard of in the last few years was the oncology advice given to a cousin of one of my best friends. Doug's cousin, a stage IV patient, asked his doctor a perfectly reasonable question: What would you do if "you were in my shoes," or words to that effect? The doctor's advice? "If I were in your shoes, I would be panicking right now." This is not a misquote.

Suffice it to say that I could keep writing on this specific topic. I have nothing but the highest respect for those who have treated me. They have each been intelligent, earnest, and hardworking, but, *most importantly*, for purposes of this section, they have been trained to think like *scientists*.

Most scientists, especially medical scientists, and especially oncologists, seem to think differently than you and I do. This is not a knock on the medical profession. As a member of the legal profession, I am acutely aware that clients can feel like lawyers have a language of their own, an all-too-common air of self-importance, and a way of thinking unique to the legal profession. Clients may occasionally feel this way about their lawyers, but I can assure you that jurors almost *never* feel this way about *successful* trial lawyers. A successful trial lawyer persuades jurors, and this means that successful trial lawyers *must* meet jurors (and clients) where they are at. This is the urgent task of any successful trial lawyer. In my experience, oncologists do not seem to feel this same sense of urgency to meet patients where they are at, and this can be attributed in large part to their scientific training.

The core gulf of communication between doctors and their patients is the gulf that exists between any scientific expert and interested layman. On this point, let me quote the best-selling author of *The Cancer Code*, Dr. Jason Fung: "Doctors and medical researchers follow the dictums of 'evidence based medicine.' The status quo is considered to be fundamentally correct, and changing that understanding requires many peer-reviewed studies."[70] Why should this be a problem? "Peer review is a search for consensus, which researchers presume is the truth. This ensures that old opinions hold and that new ideas are stifled."[71] This may seem pretty theoretical, but it's more important than you might guess, especially in the context of the principles discussed in this book.

Here, I'm going to be even a little more theoretical: the fundamental distinction between the way doctors think and the way many stage cancer patients usually think is a function of the (somewhat blurry) distinction between inductive reasoning and deductive reasoning. Inductive reasoning is essentially a bottom-up approach to reaching conclusions. Greatly simplified, inductive reasoning takes one from the specific (e.g., the scientific data as described by Dr. Fung above) to a general conclusion. Inductive reasoning is used in the search for patterns based on trained observation. Again, greatly simplified, deductive reasoning is what most people are far more used to, and engage in , every day of their lives. Deductive reasoning is akin to top-down reasoning and starts with a conclusion or hypothesis.

Let's outline this distinction with a specific example. You have just been diagnosed with stage IV NSCLC. By happenstance, you learn that a person in your circle of acquaintances, a three-year survivor no less, had the same diagnosis. This obviously piques your curiosity. After being given this person's phone number, you call him, introduce yourself and your condition, and ask him for any advice he might have for the person in your shoes. His response? "High-dose vitamin C," and then he gives a brief description of how this type of treatment helped him. You have now talked to a three-year survivor of stage IV NSCLC (he is in the roughly 15 percent survival rate category), and he is a strong advocate for high-dose vitamin C, especially during chemotherapy.

He claims it was a game changer. Best of all, he tells you one of the best high-dose vitamin clinics in the country has an office within twenty miles of your home. Having understood that you are a sample size, or n of 1, you conclude—based on this recommendation and by use of everyday, commonsense reasoning—that it makes sense to at least *try* high-dose vitamin C. This is rather exciting, is it not? All things being equal, why *wouldn't* you follow up on this survivor's advice?

At your next meeting with your oncologist, you mention this anecdote and ask what he thinks of high-dose vitamin C. Your oncologist greets *your* enthusiasm with, ahem, something less than enthusiasm, if not disdain.

He begrudgingly admits that high-dose vitamin C will "probably do no harm if you insist on doing this," but he offers a cautionary note that the vitamin C has to be "high quality" and then transitions to the role of financial counselor by expressing an opinion about the expense of such treatments. Because you are a budding rebel and plan to actually *survive*, however, you press a little harder. Why not? Why shouldn't I take high-dose vitamin C? His response is that the data have not really shown efficacy in terms of survival rates, and so on. You then press the final point: Does he recommend *against* the use of high-dose vitamin C? No, he just doesn't think it will be all that helpful. [Full disclosure: this is a sanitized version of a conversation I actually had with one of my oncologists.]

What is going on here? Is your oncologist *trying* to be a wet blanket? Is he lazy? To both questions, I would honestly say no.

Your oncologist is simply betraying the way he has been taught to *think*. "Evidence-based medicine" is the "process of systematically finding, appraising, and using contemporaneous research in the basis for clinical decisions."[72] Anecdotes do not seem to mean the same thing to you and me as they do to oncologists. Anecdotes are not data. And anecdata—a broad array of anecdotes—do not fare much better. You, on the other hand, have been told by a survivor how he believes he managed to survive chemotherapy, if not thrive while being poisoned. You see no reason to reject this hypothesis based on what you have heard. This is very exciting, yes?

Apparently, not to your oncologist. If it isn't peer-reviewed, don't expect your oncologist to find your suggestions to be all that exciting.

o o o

In your newly undertaken role of self-doctor and citizen-scientist, it is going to be important that you learn how to communicate with your oncologist in a way that ensures that you—and you alone—determine treatment strategies for Phase Two and beyond. It is entirely possible that some of those strategies will fall on either deaf or dismissive ears. It is also possible that your traditional oncologist will have a knee-jerk reaction to any strategy for cancer survival that falls outside of the accepted confines of chemotherapy, radiation, or surgery.

Am I being unfair to oncologists here? Am I painting with too broad a brush?

Let's explore this topic with a simple question: Has your oncologist suggested *any* alternative treatments that you might pursue in tandem with traditional treatments? I didn't think so.

Except in unusual cases, traditional oncologists just don't seem to think that way. Traditional oncologists seem to be highly disposed to inside-the-box treatments, and that box is a prescribed standard of care that very nearly *prevents* them from considering that there is anything useful for cancer survival *outside of that box.* Anything outside that box seems like a Hail Mary pass to traditional oncologists. That's just the way it is. This is not a moral failing by your doctor. It is a paradigm issue about how doctors and patients think about survival. Accept it. Don't get frustrated by it.

o o o

That is also why you—and you alone—must be the builder of the box. You must learn to self-doctor because you are an n of 1. You must become a citizen-scientist because it is your life on the line, and sometimes, when the clock seems to be running short, the best play in the book is indeed a Hail Mary. This is what notorious survivors do, whether they be Jackie Boggs, Glenn Sabin, Ross Douthat, or the survivors we have already met or will be meeting throughout the remainder of this book.

To sum up, there is no need for inside the box thinking to dominate during Phase Two, and, in my experience, the best route outside the box is via the route afforded by complementary alternative medicine, the subject of the next chapter.

Chapter 12: *Weighing the Possibilities of Complementary Medicine*

When it comes to chronic illness, both Western and alternative medicine read the body of the patient metaphorically. Western medicine is based on one kind of metaphor—the body is a car, its parts need upkeep, piece by piece. It is not a metaphor that works well for chronically ill patients, whose parts cannot be "fixed." Alternative medicine offers a more appealing metaphor: the body is an ecosystem and caring for it as a whole—making the patient feel seen—is crucial.

—MEGHAN O'ROURKE, *The Invisible Kingdom*

WE HAVE SPENT A FAIR AMOUNT OF TIME DISCUSSING COMMUNICA-tions with your oncologist because this is an important issue in and of itself. And as others and I have emphasized, *you* are in charge of your healing, and you cannot allow yourself to be hampered in this process by gulfs in communication, dogmatic dismissals, or the temptation of the roads most traveled. You are truly an n of 1.

This leads us to a discussion of complementary medicine. Among cancer survivors, two out of three reportedly have used some form of complementary and alternative medicine (CAM). 43 percent of those survivors have reportedly used CAM within the prior twelve months.[73] The previous chapters' discussions about communication, self-doctoring, and thinking styles are also important as they relate to CAM.

If you peruse Amazon, for instance, you are going to find a deluge of books written by cancer patients and cancer advocates about alternative treatments, with a large subset of those focusing on diet and other holistic alternatives. I have referred to some of these books in earlier pages. This chapter is going to discuss two of the primary alternative treatments I have consistently pursued since my diagnosis. I understand alternative treatments tend not to be covered by health insurance. I am also aware that the typical stage IV cancer patient does not have limitless funds set aside for what I have termed "parallel silo" treatments. But here I will repeat the line I used with my integrative oncologist, Dr. Lucas Tims, when I first met him and he outlined a recommended course of treatment for me in January 2020: "Well, I've been saving thirty years for a rainy day, and it is certainly raining right now."

Only you know whether to pursue and how to afford CAM treatments. And unfortunately, only you can decide which alternative treatments make sense *for you*. With that caveat, let me outline why I chose the parallel silo treatments of acupuncture and high-dose vitamin C as my particular complementary medicine options during the past five years.

o o o

Let's first talk about acupuncture. "Approximately one in 10 cancer survivors have used acupuncture in the United States."[74]

Acupuncture is a staple of traditional Chinese medicine and has been a healing strategy for almost three thousand years. Thin needles are inserted into the body with the goal of balancing the flow of energy or life force, sometimes called Chi. As a martial artist in an Okinawan tradition, I found the notions of Chi or energy meridians fairly intuitive. Thus, I was not thrown off by the basic theory behind acupuncture. It helps that those needles do not generally bother me.

I have had approximately seventy-five acupuncture treatments since my diagnosis. Whenever possible, I scheduled an acupuncture treatment the *day before* my chemotherapy treatment. I was fairly religious about this, and I truly believe this allowed me to survive and thrive during most of my chemotherapy treatments. The treatments are basically about an hour. My particular acupuncturist specializes in cancer patients and has an outstanding reputation. As a prelude to each treatment, he would listen to and "read" my pulse, and then in went the needles. I used that intervening forty-five or so minutes to meditate. Fairly simple and not all that expensive. And I met a new, very good friend.

But did it *truly* help?

In my experience the answer is yes. I certainly had my butt kicked by chemotherapy, especially the second regimen, after my recurrence. *But* I never lost my hair, I continued to read avidly and play golf, and people were generally surprised to know when they learned I had been diagnosed with stage IV lung cancer, let alone a recurrence and a second cancer. I attribute a contributing factor in this outcome to acupuncture.

But what is the "scientific" answer to the question?

The scientific research in this area is actually quite robust and has gathered steam in the past twenty years. I will not try to summarize all of it here, but the bottom line is that acupuncture is a strong parallel silo of treatment in helping you survive chemotherapy with *very little, if any*, downside. For instance, a recent systematic review and meta-analysis suggests that "acupuncture may be an effective intervention to reduce pain associated with cancer."[75] As a curious citizen-scientist, it is highly likely that you will be able to access reliable scientific information on any other questions you may have in connection with acupuncture, and its relation to your cancer treatments.

I highly recommend your consideration of acupuncture in conjunction with your lung cancer treatments, but you should check with your traditional oncologist before undertaking such treatments. For me, acupuncture was a core parallel silo of treatment, and at a minimum, acupuncture may help you survive your treatments while helping you keep your hair.

o o o

I have already sung the praises of integrative oncologists. What I haven't specifically done is discuss the role of high-dose vitamins, and in particular, high-dose vitamin C, in conjunction with your conventional cancer treatments. High-dose intravenously administered vitamin C (IVC) is "widely used in cancer patients by complementary and alternative medicine practitioners."[76]

Since my diagnosis, I have received at least seventy-five high-dose vitamin C treatments. These treatments were usually administered in conjunction with the timing of my chemotherapy treatments and were, in my opinion, instrumental in helping me to survive my traditional cancer treatments. Again, as is the case with acupuncture, there is a great deal of publicly available research at your disposal regarding the efficacy of high-dose vitamins in cancer treatments. I strongly recommend that you review this research and consider whether this parallel silo will aid you in your cancer survival.

o o o

The bottom line when it comes to CAM is that because complementary medicine is generally not cheap, one must be judicious about which CAM strategy is pursued. I also believe these strategies should not be pursued absent a consultation with an integrative oncologist. I have given you some ideas of what has helped me. You must now determine, in your role as self-doctor and citizen-scientist, what will help you.

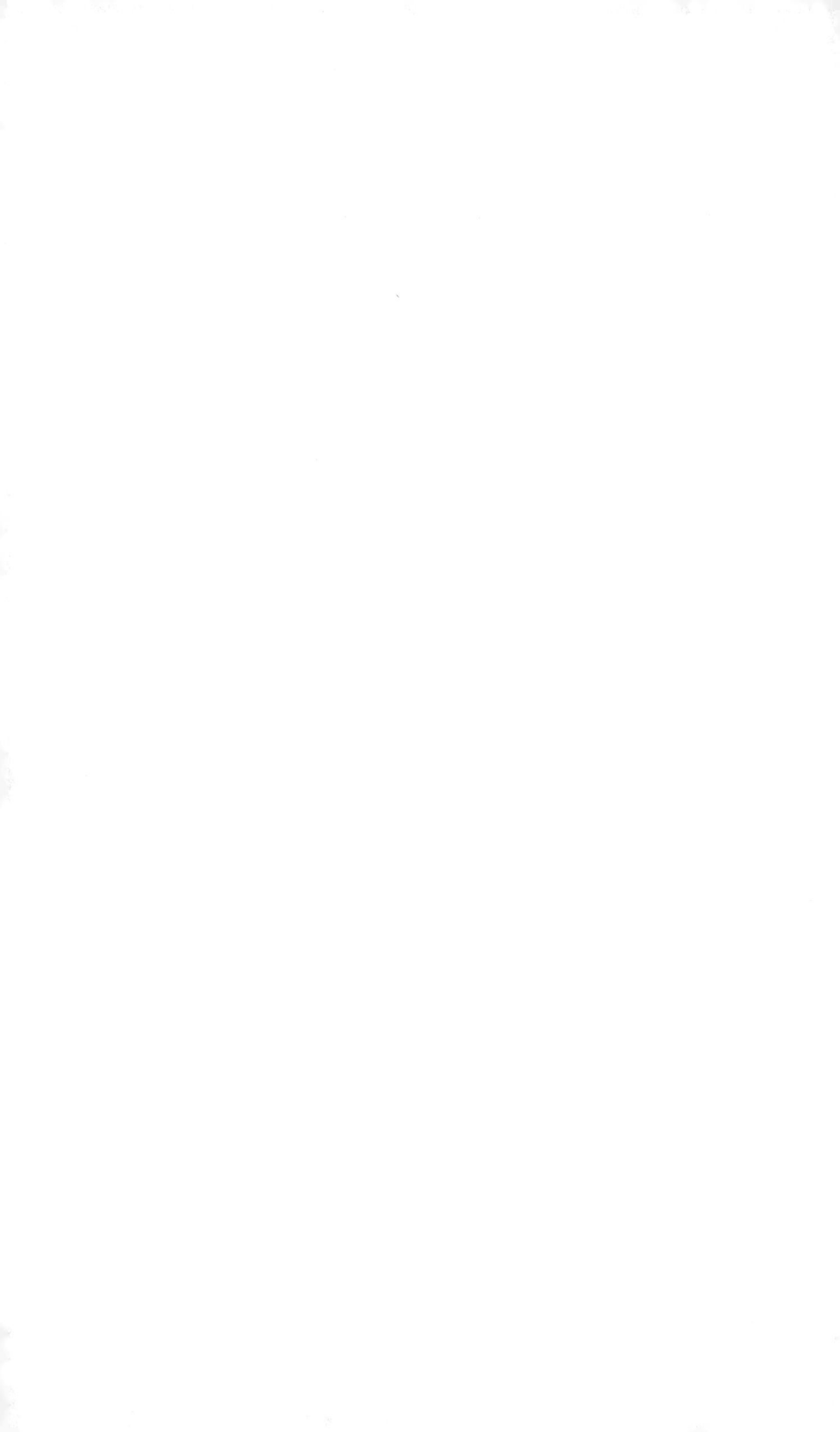

Chapter 13: *Navigating the Mental Game of Scans*

Scan-associated distress is a common problem among patients with NSCLC, and is associated with impaired quality of life.

—Joshua M. Bauml, MD, *Lung Cancer Journal*, August 16, 2016

In the first year after your diagnosis, you are likely to have several scans to gauge the progress of your treatments. The days leading up to such scans are quite stressful. The waiting game in the hours after such scans is even more stressful. The common term for this stress is called "scanxiety."

I would like to claim that I have figured out how to deal with these stressors, but alas, I'm afraid there does not seem to be a magic bullet here either. Scanxiety happens. Scanxiety *is*. The question is: How might one lessen its severity?

If you are like me, you don't really worry about scans until about a week or so before the upcoming appointment. No cancer survivor I know of worries about scans each and every day between appointments. So here is the mental game technique I have used for a rapidly approaching scan: I simply remind myself that there is nothing that can be done about the outcome. In other words, by the time the date of the upcoming scan and its concomitant anxiety approaches, I remind myself that the die is cast, so to speak. If the die is cast, then there really is nothing to be done. And if there is nothing to be done, what is there to be anxious about? This is an approach to quite literally accepting something in real time—what "I cannot change." Simple, but not easy.

In the midst of writing this chapter, I decided to test my own advice in the days before a recent scan. This was my second scan after the completion of radiation for the lung cancer recurrence. In some ways, this was the second-most important scan of the previous four years, apart from the initial scan that led to my NSCLC diagnosis. As the upcoming scan began to approach, I began to suffer some of the "usual" anxiety about what might happen. Then I reminded myself of the advice I am offering in this chapter. I reminded myself that there was very little or nothing I could do to affect the outcome of the scan. This created a remarkable sense of calm. I knew the die was already cast. There was nothing to be anxious about. I can tell you from experience that this approach works if you give it a chance to work.

There is truly no secret remedy available or offered here to those who must endure the eve and the wake of their scans. If my earlier advice has resonated with you, you may perhaps have already visualized the outcome of a good scan. If the scan is less than favorable, you will simply have to use the information and experiences you have already acquired to assess the appropriate plan of action.

Scans are an opportunity for you, once again, to develop what Gonzales calls a "frank relationship with risk, which is the essence of life."[77] Is the forty-eight-hour window before and after a scan stressful? Yes, it is. By the time your anxiety and the date of that scan approaches is there anything you can do to affect the outcome? Probably not.

My simple advice is a modified form of advice offered by our friends, the Stoics. As Seneca said, "He suffers more than necessary, who suffers before it is necessary."[78] Put another way, try not to add to the suffering inherent in battling cancer by being anxious about an event that, by the time your scan approaches, is outside of your control.

Chapter 14: *Weighing the Potential of Diets, Fasting, and Supplements*

Fructose appears to be able to directly fuel not only colon cancer but cancers of the breast, lung, and pancreas. ... If you want to make cancer happy, feed it fructose.

—RICHARD JOHNSON, quoted in Sam Apple's *Ravenous*

THE FINAL PHASE TWO ISSUE I WISH TO ADDRESS IS THE QUESTIONS of diet, fasting, and supplements.

Let's start with the subject of diets. People seem to get quite worked up about diets in the cancer world. My guess is that I have received more unsolicited advice about "diet" in the past five years than any other subject, and not just from the vegans and erstwhile hippies either. All of it is well-meaning, if a little presumptuous. To reiterate, I have surmised that there must be a strong subconscious factor in play when a never-smoker gets lung cancer. Lung cancer is associated so much with smoking that a type of cognitive dissonance develops among friends and family when a never-smoker gets this disease. And among a certain subset of friends and family, the discomfort created by this cognitive dissonance seems to be alleviated by diet advice.

Kelly Turner's book *Radical Remission*, which I have pillaged throughout these pages for insight, quotes, and wisdom, has a subtitle about cancer diets called "No Sweets, No Meats, No Dairy, No

Refined Foods."[79] This seems like a pretty catchy rule of thumb. Full disclosure: for me, this rule of thumb lasted about two days.

Having reviewed this subject in some detail and having discussed this topic with those I respect greatly, I have not been persuaded that one's particular diet significantly matters in getting or surviving cancer. I harken back to my friend's eight-month-old daughter in chemotherapy: Did baby Eliza not pursue the right diet in her first eight months of life? I also harken to one of my best friend's daughter Liesel, who, at fifteen years old, died of stage IV cancer, as did her mother, Courtney, roughly three years later. Both Liesel and Courtney pursued extremely healthy diets before and during their cancer treatments. Were these diets to blame for their cancers or their having not survived? Nobody of sober mind would claim this, nor does any reasonable scientific evidence support such a claim.

Remember: when it comes to diet, here, too, *you are an n of 1*.

Regarding *my* personal science experiment, I was advised by conventional oncologists that no particular diet was called for during any of my treatments, and although I didn't necessarily believe that all diets were equal, I also was not too thrilled about the prospect of eating like a rabbit, a hermit, or an Olympic athlete. I have tried to eat a relatively strict Keto diet—more off than on—because such a diet appeared to me to potentially reduce inflammation, the data seemed comparatively convincing, and the results at least correlated with my feeling markedly better. I have also restricted all sweets (fructose) fairly dramatically, not because of great self-discipline but mainly because I don't really like sweets all that much anyway.

It seems pretty intuitive to me that if the equivalent of sugar is used to get the attention of cancer in PET scans, it's probably not a great idea for a person with any type of stage IV cancer to eat too many candy bars or desserts. As leading cancer researcher Richard Johnson says, "If you want to make cancer happy, feed it fructose."[80] Traditional oncologists do not seem to agree with this fairly basic reasoning, but there are leading cancer researchers who do. For instance, Lewis Cantley, "the scientist who pioneered the study of how insulin activates the pathways linked to cancer," is convinced that sugar is linked to cancer.[81] In fact, Cantley "has stopped eating sugar himself for a simple reason. His research has led him to the conclusion that today's high consumption of sugar is 'almost certainly responsible for the increased rates of cancers in the developed world.'"[82] The same principles are true of alcohol consumption, which, since my diagnosis, has not been an issue.

o o o

There are amazing and well-sourced books that discuss the "correct" diet for cancer patients. I especially enjoyed *The Metabolic Approach to Cancer*, which not only favors a keto diet but also gives a very powerful discussion of the general topic of cancer and the specific limitations of conventional medical treatments.[83] The clincher for me, however, was once again Dr. Fung's *The Cancer Code*: diet *may* matter, but science hasn't really figured out *which* diet matters *the most*. So, my position, which not coincidentally fits my general disdain for the discussion of diet in the context of cancer, is that there are other fish to fry, so to speak.[84]

I have also been committed to the concept of intermittent fasting, the efficacy of which is developing a pretty sound scientific consensus, especially in enhancing chemotherapy. Briefly, intermittent fasting is the intentional skipping of one or more meals. The idea is to jolt your body and immune system. I typically do not eat after about 8:00 p.m., and I generally skip breakfast. I rarely eat three meals on any given day. This gives my body somewhere in the neighborhood of sixteen hours when it is in a "fasting" state. The scientific research on the efficacy of intermittent fasting is quite robust as well.[85]

As I write this, I weigh less than I have weighed in the past twenty years. Some of this can be attributed to the side effects of getting five separate parts of my body radiated in the past eighteen months, so that could easily change in the next six months. But I have also stayed active, playing regular rounds of golf, I have decently managed my weight, and I have also undertaken intentional exercise regimens.

You are close to the mark if you are sensing my ambivalence on this topic. I'm not telling you to put away your juicer. Just don't ask me to drink your smoothies. My overall diet advice is that if you do not possess the indifference on this subject that I cannot seem to shake, pick a reasonable diet and stick with it. Experiment with fasting, especially intermittent fasting. Fortune favors the bold, and the placebo effect is your friend.[86] Such actions will, at a minimum, help keep unneeded weight off and reduce obesity, a known risk factor in your fight with cancer.[87]

If, like me, you have no appetite for diets, don't let the perfect be the enemy of the good: at least endeavor to minimize your consumption of the obvious culprits: sugar and alcohol.

o o o

Over-the-counter supplements are your friend if they do not interfere with the effectiveness of your conventional treatments. Why? "The main difference between chemotherapy and vitamin or herbal supplements is that most chemotherapy is designed to kill cancer cells, while most supplements are designed to strengthen the immune system so that *it* can then remove cancer cells."[88] In other words, supplements help your immune system.

I think it is important for a cancer patient to have a *formal* assessment of the need for dietary supplements. I received this assessment from my integrative oncologist, who made recommendations after a series of targeted screenings. Assuming you have access to and can afford the advice of an integrative oncologist, there is no need for you to figure out the question of supplements on your own. An integrative oncologist can also help to ensure that no supplement you take might interfere with any other treatments you are undertaking.

As for particular supplements, there is clearly strong evidence that turmeric has powerful anti-cancer properties. This is confirmed by a variety of sources.[89] You should seriously consider this particular nutritional supplement. Here, I will also suggest for your consideration a dietary supplement called Salvestrols. Salvestrols are a dietary supplement that, in effect, provide the benefits of organic fruits and vegetables. There is a reasonably robust body of research to support their enlistment as a cancer-fighting supplement, including for lung cancer specifically.[90] I have been taking Salvestrols for more than three years.

o o o

By the time you are well into Phase Two, you are now a well-practiced self-doctor and citizen-scientist. You also, I hope, appreciate the importance of parallel silos of cancer treatments. Even a minimally exploratory Google search is likely to bombard you with information about cancer diets, fasting, and supplements. Listen to your intuition. Do your own research. Dig below the surface. Get outside your comfort zone. Then, make a decision about diets, fasting, and supplements and stick to that decision while paradoxically keeping an open mind about what works and what doesn't work.

This is responsible hope in action.

PART III

Resilient Hope—Surviving Years Two through Five

Within this or that framework of viewing life, cancer is still a significant adversity. But people do build resilience if they are granted the right conditions.

—MORHAF AL ACHKAR, MD, PhD, *Roads to Meaning and Resilience with Cancer*

I am a fellow cancer patient doing all I can to learn from my disease and change my life because of it. I am gravely ill, yet weirdly well. More grateful to my cancer than afraid of it. Inhabiting a rarified space between my fierce will to live and my necessary willingness to die.

—SOPHIE SABBAGE, *The Cancer Whisperer*

Chapter 15: *Understanding the Importance of Resilient Hope*

Interestingly, despite substantial distress that is associated with a cancer diagnosis and its treatment, many cancer patients manifest remarkable resilience.

—"Resilience in Cancer Patients," *Front Psychiatry* 10 (2019): 208

THE OXFORD DICTIONARY DEFINITION OF RESILIENCE IS "THE capacity to withstand or to recover quickly from difficulties; toughness." Toughness is a word that resonates here. Resilience is a *capacity*, akin to a muscle, capable of development and refinement. Resilient hope is what is required during Phase Three, and this capacity is built from and then refined by the "push" and the "pull" capacities already developed in Phases One and Two.

Unless you are quite lucky, the capacity for resilient hope is likely to be tested in Phase Three of your NSCLC survival. In my experience, this capacity was tested quite starkly by a second cancer, notwithstanding some of the bravado I have already described. I remember being distinctly *shaken*, not so much by having prostate cancer (most men over the age of fifty have either active or inactive prostate cancer), but—at least initially—by the notion that the anticancer strategies I had been pursuing had "failed." Or so I thought for a short time. The time limit I placed on whining about the unfairness of having developed prostate cancer was two weeks after diagnosis, although Rebecca might remember an additional week or two was tacked on during that unfortunate summer.

I was also shaken by my NSCLC recurrence, which was diagnosed not long after I had thrown away the unused catheters associated with the prostate cancer treatments. The recurrence was not necessarily a *new* testing ground for resilience, but it was a testing ground, nevertheless. Nothing fundamentally changes with a second cancer or with a recurrence. They are simply new "events" on the survival horizon, and the same principles we have been discussing apply: rebel, take responsibility, look to the role models, stoke that energy we are calling the will to live, and, yes, especially in Phase Three, develop the capacity called resilient hope.

The bottom line is that you are likely to be tested again in Phase Three. Building resilient hope in this phase is the move from intermediate-level cancer survival to advanced-level cancer survival. Consider Phase Three to be your chance to add to your arsenal of cancer survival strategies and to refine the strategies you have already developed. And keep this in mind: From a survival rate standpoint, to use the words of Laurence Gonzales, you are already one of the "notorious" ones. You know what you are doing. This is a cause for celebration.

Chapter 16: *Setting Realistic Goals—Metastases and Quiescence*

In cancer treatment, the gold medal is finding out that the tumors are shrinking. Silver—and who wouldn't want a silver medal?—is that you are stable. There is no bronze.

> —Caitlin Flanagan, "I Thought Stage IV Cancer Was Bad Enough," *The Atlantic*, June 2020

To survive a stage IV NSCLC diagnosis the first year or longer, what specifically is *required*? What specific goal should you be working toward or visualizing?

One might think that eradicating *all* cancer from your body is a good start. And in the general cancer world, this sometimes happens. This is generally referred to as "no evidence of disease," which means that no cancer is detectable within the observatory powers of your latest scan. As I have mentioned, when I was treated for laser ablation on my prostate, my oncologist, in effect, "spot-welded" the cancerous cells from my prostate. This was a state-of-the-art technique and, given the limited nature of my prostate cancer, was entirely feasible. The cancer is indeed currently absent from my latest scan.

Unfortunately, "no evidence of disease" is not a realistically probable expectation for those with advanced NSCLC lung cancer. Let me repeat an important line from the 2020 NSCLC Study:

"None of the patients surviving 10 years were disease free, which is not surprising since all of the patients had stage IV disease at the beginning of the study." Again: *none* of the long term, AWD survivors were "disease free."[91] Not a lot of play in those joints.

In my legal career, I have had to deal with thousands of witnesses, whether in depositions, on the witness stand, or in informal interviews. There is a pretty good rule of thumb about witnesses: not a single one of them is perfect. Every witness has warts, even the "expert" witnesses. I have never once called a witness to the witness stand and had them escape without getting hit by the other side. After dozens of these experiences, I adopted a rule of thumb about witnesses and repeated it *ad nauseam* to my trial colleagues: "Don't let the perfect be the enemy of the good." In other words—no irony intended here—every witness is going to take some lumps.

o o o

This same principle applies to surviving cancer: when formulating your specific goals for survival, don't let the perfect be the enemy of the good.

Absent a spontaneous healing or miracle cure, you are not likely to entirely *eradicate* from your body the cancer that led to your stage IV diagnosis. Placed in proper context, this is actually what I think my MD Anderson oncologist *meant* when, in our first meeting, and after she sensed that I was being just a bit too optimistic about my treatments, her body language and her demeanor changed. She then looked at me very directly and said, "I don't know if anybody has told you this yet, but I feel like I should tell you this. There is no cure for your condition."

This was about four to five weeks after my initial diagnosis. I did not have the tools then that I have now to understand what she was *really* saying—not that I was destined to die sometime soon from this disease, but that given the best medicine available in 2020, it was highly unlikely that my treatments would permanently eradicate all cancer from my right lung, lymph nodes, and spine.

Can survivors actually *survive* because the metastasis that led originally to the stage IV diagnosis has died down? The answer is yes. The cancer has not been *cured*: the cancerous cells have stopped dividing. They have become stable or quiescent.

The term "quiescent" is a term my MD Anderson oncologist introduced in the same conversation I described above. By way of context, we had been discussing whether a biopsy was needed to test for genetic mutations. She was concerned about doing another biopsy—this would have been my third biopsy in less than six weeks—because she had determined, by reviewing my various scans over the past thirty to forty days, that the cancer seemed to be "quiescent."

Of course, I had to google this term to make sure it was as good as it sounded. *Quiescent* means "in a state of inactivity or dormancy." When I experienced a recurrence about thirty months after our initial consultation, this same oncologist used this term again and actually seemed pleased that—notwithstanding the recurrence—my particular cancer was a "slow" cancer. Even in recurrence, the cancer had not spread to any new sites, with the exception of a possible spot in my left lung. Instead, several of the original offending lymph nodes and the same spot on my spine had "lit up." She also seemed to think this was, in context, good news.

What is the upshot of all of this? The upshot is that—given that you are a stage IV NSCLC patient—you should not so much worry about cancer eradication as *cancer quiescence*. Or, to put it another way, the goal is to keep metastases at bay.

○ ○ ○

Metastasis, *and the halting of it*, is the name of the game in Phase Two, Three, and beyond. More to the point, metastasis is responsible for 90 percent of all cancer deaths.[92] A given cancerous tumor or lesion can be benign or malignant and, thus, identical "except that benign cancers lack...metastatic activity and cause almost no significant disease."[93] Again, as you now know, that which is termed "advanced" cancer is not necessarily terminal cancer: advanced cancer is cancer that has "advanced" beyond its otherwise dormant stage and then has spread. The key with your treatments and other strategies is *not only* to kill as many of those cancer cells as possible but, ultimately, to halt *metastases* as well.

In Phase Three and beyond, it is important to have realistic goals. You are not likely to have the fortune of a miracle cure. The spread and reduction of cancer should be your primary concern. It is metastases that "makes cancer more lethal than any other disease in existence."[94] Halting metastases is a realistic and worthy goal, and may be the "secret" of cancer.[95]

Let me add one more element to the equation: don't let dreams of the perfect (a miracle cure) be the enemy of the good (quiescence). Gratefully accept that gold or silver prize, enjoy such times of stability on the long path of surviving cancer, and try not to burden yourself with unrealistic expectations. Remember the words of Caitlin Flanagan quoted above: no bronze prizes are awarded.

Chapter 17: *Navigating the Paradox of Double Mind*

The absorbing fact about being mortally sick is that you spend a good deal of time preparing yourself to die ... while simultaneously and highly interested in the business of survival.

—CHRISTOPHER HITCHENS, *Mortality*

IT'S TIME TO GET PHILOSOPHICAL AGAIN, WHICH MAY SEEM unnecessary, but here again the words of Laurence Gonzales are apt: "If you want to be a survivor, be a philosopher."[96]

Surviving cancer can sometimes be as simple as gaining a comfort level with the idea of paradox. In Phase One, you must learn to push *against*—to reject conventional wisdom while also understanding it deeply. In Phase Two, you must learn to pull *within*, to embrace personal responsibility for your health while also being administered fairly deadly treatments by third parties. In Phase Three, you very likely will be presented with the opportunity to learn how to do both of these actions at once, but with the benefit of an experienced survivor's hard-won perspective.

These paradoxes are likely to present themselves at a more deeply philosophical level. We discussed earlier the transition of my home office from a "war room" to a "peace room." My sense is that there is likely a time when every stage IV cancer patient must make a mental transition of this kind, and Phase Three is a time frame ripe for this transition. The transition is from a "war footing" to something akin to a "peace footing." The need for this transition becomes more apparent, at least in my experience, with the passage of time and seems to present itself somewhere around a year or so after diagnosis.

∘ ∘ ∘

My intuitive sense of the need for this transition was heightened as I began to take more notice of friends and acquaintances with cancer in the year or so after my diagnosis. There is the classic cliché that once one decides to buy, say, a red Camaro, all one sees on the road are red Camaros. Something like this, but quite unfortunate, happens in the cancer context as well. Once I had been diagnosed, I was struck by how many others in my circle of friends and acquaintances were also dealing with cancer. Some of these friends and acquaintances were suffering quite acutely from their cancer treatments. Observing this seemed to instigate the reflections I am describing.

The passage of time periodically provided stark reminders in a different way, a way that accelerated the transition from war to peace: far too many of those friends and acquaintances were *dying* of cancer. As a conservative estimate, I am personally aware of at least a dozen friends and acquaintances who have died of cancer since my original diagnosis. The age range of this group is widely disparate, from fifteen-year-old Liesel, who I have already mentioned, to a golf buddy in his sixties named Duke. A very close high school friend of my wife, Denise, also died in this time frame. She became one of my closest cancer friends, and she was the person who turned me on to acupuncture. Another one of the individuals I met with, Sean, who looked great, had a very positive attitude, and seemed to be doing quite well surviving stage III skin cancer. He died just a few months after we met. The list goes on, unfortunately. I am sure you could compile such a list as well.

As these deaths and recurrences started to accumulate, my feeling of being on a war footing waned. I began to embrace the more nuanced notion of acceptance instead: I was no longer so intensely interested in fighting cancer; I was more inclined to accept that cancer was a part of my life, that, yes, I planned to survive, and that this chronic disease needed to be *managed*. Acceptance brought more peace. Not only was my cancer quiescent during a fair portion of this time, so too was my outlook.

o   o   o

There is indeed a paradox here. On the one hand, one must fight because the war is not even close to over. On the other hand, if we are being honest, one gets tired of fighting—physically tired of it—and one certainly gets tired of the war. The words I quoted to begin this chapter of famed and prolific author Christopher Hitchens, who died not so long ago of esophageal cancer, explains this paradox, and are worth quoting again: "The absorbing fact about being mortally sick is that you spend a good deal of time preparing yourself to die with some modicum of stoicism (and provision for loved ones), while simultaneously and highly interested in the business of survival."[97] Is this paradox *easy* to navigate? No. Again, the words of Hitchens: "This is a distinctly bizarre way of 'living'—lawyers in the morning and doctors in the afternoon—*and means one has to exist even more than usual in a double frame of mind*"[98] (emphasis added).

This is not unique to survivors in the cancer setting. This is a common characteristic of survival in every setting. Laurence Gonzales calls this paradox "active passiveness," the ability to accept the situation one is in "without giving into it."[99] Active passiveness is, in fact, a recognized spiritual principle of the highest order.[100]

Yes, surviving cancer is a distinctly bizarre way of living.

How does one navigate this "double frame of mind"? How does one adopt a posture of acceptance while in the midst of a fight? In my experience, this is a more practical question than one might think. We are now discussing Phase Three of cancer survival, years two through five. You have been fighting cancer for at least one year and probably longer. The "four-alarm-fire" element of survival seems to have died down. But has it, *in fact*, died down? As a matter of fact, the fire has most assuredly *not* died down.

The numbers related to survival rates have not really changed. Consistently, with each anniversary of one's diagnosis date, the numbers in Phase Three are not materially different than they were in Phases One or Two, that is, roughly 70 percent of the patient population survives into each subsequent phase, with what I have outlined as nice uptick in survival probability for those that reach the fifth anniversary of their diagnosis. I am not being pessimistic (or optimistic) here, but brutally factual.

o o o

One cannot live life in a constant state of war, but one can do what is possible to prevent war, or to be prepared for war, or to survive that war when it comes again. If you have survived more than a year with what is considered "terminal" cancer, you have likely—perhaps subconsciously—learned to navigate the paradox of war and peace. Now is the time to *consciously* develop this strategy.

The core of any such strategy is vigilance. I began this chapter discussing the seemingly persistent reminder that develops as others around you are suffering from or even dying from cancer. Each of these people is a reminder to be vigilant, to not let one's guard down. Each of these people is also a reminder that you might have something to offer others diagnosed with cancer, a subject addressed in a subsequent chapter. Maintain a war footing, in other words, but live in peace. Learn to occupy that "rarified space" between the "fierce will to live and [a] necessary willingness to die."[101]

On the one hand, it seems that we must "fight" with all our might, even in Phases Two, Three, and beyond. But, on the other hand, surrender, acceptance, and peace within the "rarified space" occupied by cancer survivors also have their place. Everybody must navigate this paradox in their own way. I do not struggle too much with this ambiguity, but I also admit that I am not really offering much for you to hang your hat on here.

o o o

In Phase One, we must summon our warrior energy and declare total war on cancer. We push against conventional wisdom. In Phase Two, we take ownership of our healing and pull the responsibility for healing inward. In the subsequent Phases of cancer survival, however, there is a place for active passiveness—something akin to "peace through strength."

As we will learn in the next chapter, the paradox may even develop in us a new purpose for our lives.

Chapter 18: *Taking Advantage of Remission*

What does it mean for a chronically ill patient to heal? In some cases, it may mean a remission of disease. But in others, it means the patient is now able to manage the illness with some degree of integrity.
—MEGHAN O'ROURKE, *The Invisible Kingdom*

LUNG CANCER IS CONSIDERED TO BE IN REMISSION "WHEN A patient has fewer or no symptoms and the doctors can see that the cancer has shrunk or vanished on imaging scans."[102] This standard applies to NSCLC as well.

Somewhere in the midst of a series of "good" scans about a year after my diagnosis, I asked my primary oncologist the question: "Am I in remission?" I was being a little crafty. I already knew the answer. In my role as citizen-scientist, I had done some homework. I knew my cancer was stable—certainly worthy of the silver medal referred to by Caitlin Flanagan earlier—and that it could be said that I was technically in remission. Most relevant of all, however, I knew that the term was only useful, if at all, until my next scan. So, what was my doctor's answer to this loaded question? He said my cancer was "stable" and indicated a distinct preference not to discuss the subject further. I let it go at that.

The answer I was given was similar, at least in principle, to the question I was asked by every client on the eve of every case I ever tried. Are we going to win the case? The answer to both questions? It depends. If a lawyer ever tells you that you have, say, a "70 percent" chance of winning an upcoming case, you might want to ask for his bar card or, less directly, ask him to clarify his response. What he probably means is that if your case were tried to a jury ten times, you would probably win the case seven of those ten times. But that also means you would lose three of those times. That's why the actual outcome of any specific trial is always the same: *it depends.*

This same principle applies to discussions of maintaining any period of remission. It depends. It depends on your next scan. Your doctor, if she is being forthright, cannot tell you how long your remission or stable condition will last. You will be asked by friends or acquaintances every once in a while whether you are "in remission." There is no harm in saying yes to this question if that is the case. But, again, "remission" is just a word, a word that quickly evaporates when you least expect it. Part of resilient hope is having a straightforward understanding of what doctors can and cannot predict. Another element of resilient hope is knowing that many of the words used in the cancer world are either euphemisms or conceptual constructs, pending the outcome of your next scan.

o o o

Whether one chooses to use the word *remission* or "stable" to describe the period after a successful round of treatments is not important. What *is* important is that you take advantage of such periods. "It is a part of the natural cycle of human emotion to let down your guard once you've reached your goal."[103] The temptation will be to return to your former life in some way, and this comfortable approach is certainly understandable. But you are not the same person who was first diagnosed. Heraclitus said that "nobody steps into the same river twice." He intended a double meaning here—neither you *nor* the river are the same.

After my first round of treatments, and after the cancer had stabilized, a recurring intuition would present itself: "Don't squander this." I knew I had just dodged a bullet, so implicit in this recurrent thought was the idea that *now* was the time to move forward with a life that included a chronic disease. I was not going to wait around for my next scan but seek out new opportunities that accounted for my disease but that weren't driven by that disease. To use Caitlin Flanagan's terminology, I knew it was important to enjoy my silver medal—who wouldn't want a silver medal?—but also understood a silver medal is not necessarily a permanent award. The shiny medal could be taken off the shelf rather abruptly. This, again, is the push and the pull of Phase Three. Enjoy your stability, but don't assume it will last forever. This requires an attitude of hopeful resilience.

Surviving beyond a year with what is considered "terminal" and one of the deadliest of cancers is a traumatic experience. But there is good news awaiting many of those who survived such experiences: "Studies have shown that overcoming cancer and its treatment can be an opportunity for personal growth, as well as for enhanced mental and emotional well-being that could potentially be linked to better coping with disease related demands."[104] Or, if I might translate: (1) cancer is traumatic; (2) once you have survived treatments, enhanced personal growth from that trauma is possible; and (3) that personal growth may very well allow you to better cope with any further cancer complications in the future.

In other words—science tells us not to squander our remission!

o   o   o

It is not my place to advise anybody on how they might engage in personal growth during periods of remission or stability. I can tell you some of the strategies I have pursued.

As you now know, one of the significant strategies has been to write a book about cancer survival, with the aim of helping others traveling this same path. The writing of this book has, itself, been a major element in my own healing and my primary avenue for taking advantage of times of remission and stability. I have also taken up oil painting in a fairly serious way. This non-cancer-related pursuit has been a source of gratification and has also allowed for a shared experience with my daughter, Jacqulyn, who has been on the cancer frontlines with Rebecca during the past five years. There have been additional avenues pursued by our family to help those dealing with cancer, including involvement in the installation of a "wall of hope" at the local cancer center where I have been treated.

I cannot tell you how to write the story of your remission or how this should play out in your life, but I do think it is important to pursue activities that embody a broader purpose or, perhaps, a reminder of just how close to the edge of the cliff you have been. "The stories we tell about illness are almost entirely about overcoming it, but for illnesses that cannot be overcome, they are about growing wiser as a result of suffering."[105]One way of "growing wiser" is resisting the temptation to live proactively *only* after a good scan. You will be tempted to put life "on hold" pending that upcoming scan in six weeks or after an upcoming checkup.

In Japanese culture, there is a term for the pursuit of such activities, even while such uncertainty is present. The term is *ichigo ichie*. My favorite translated description of this term is "in this moment, an opportunity."[106] Consider those periods of stability or remission to be your chance to employ *ichigo ichie*, to employ the wisdom you have gained by suffering and survival—to avoid deferring life's opportunities because of the uncertainty of your condition.

As with so many other areas of deep survival, listen to your inner voice about this, and then act on that inner voice.

Chapter 19: *Dealing with Recurrences and Second Cancers*

> *Recurrences and second cancers suck.*
> —PAUL D. SEYFERTH

I PROMISE THAT I SEARCHED FOR AN INSPIRING QUOTE ABOUT recurrences and second cancers to begin this chapter, but I truly couldn't find one. Alas, do we need a scientific study to demonstrate that second cancers and recurrences suck?

Recurrences happen, it seems, when you least expect them. This was certainly true in my case. The morning of the scan that resulted in a recurrence, I felt as good as I had felt since before my diagnosis. I felt especially good when I went for the scan, partly because my health and strength were as strong as any time before the original diagnosis. The recurrence felt like a form of betrayal. And I felt like I had let my family and friends down. But then it was time to get back to work.

Recurrences will test your resolve, and they certainly will test your will to live. Recurrences require the most of our resilience. Recurrences are, in some ways, worse than the initial diagnosis.

No trial lawyer ever wants to try the same case twice, especially a case with bad facts, especially a case won by barely a whisker. No cancer survivor ever wants to go through treatments again. But take heart: You are no longer new to this game. You have learned the push and pull of cancer survival. Your will to live has already been tested and found worthy of this path. If you are in Phase Two or Three or beyond, you are already one of Laurence Gonzales's notorious ones.

"In the United States, more than 8% of adults diagnosed with the most common cancers developed a second malignancy."[107] Between 30 and 55 percent of NSCLC patients experience a recurrence.[108] Some of us are presented with the improbable scenario of dealing with both. Each such instance must be dealt with on its own terms, with the added benefit of resilient hope.

o o o

Some of what follows runs the risk of repeating portions of what I have previously discussed in previous chapters. I think the risk is worth it in this context because recurrences and second cancers are, at bottom, repeat performances.

Being diagnosed with prostate cancer while in the middle of a fairly successful course of treatments for lung cancer was an excellent opportunity to apply the lessons of the previous months and years of survival. As I told my wife, prostate cancer was a very direct opportunity for me "to put my money where my mouth is." Getting a second cancer seems very unfair, but I am not going to claim this caused a dark night of the soul. I actually considered the new diagnosis somewhat comical. I was diagnosed with NSCLC thirty days before COVID hit. I went through radiation and chemotherapy in the midst of the first worldwide pandemic in almost a hundred years. Then Rebecca and I both got COVID within a week of my completing chemotherapy in late 2020. *Of course,* I picked up another cancer. Thankfully, the prostate cancer had nothing to do with the lung cancer. Prostate cancer was, in the words of one of the more personable of my phalanx of oncologists, just "really shitty luck."

Yessir, I would say that hits the mark, maybe even the bullseye. It turns out that there is an almost one-to-one relationship between one's age and the chances of having prostate cancer. I thus had a 58 percent chance of being diagnosed with prostate cancer *while also* happening to experience lung cancer. I guess the 42 percent option was not in the cards.

Thankfully, my experience with lung cancer made the assessment of treatment options for prostate cancer rather straightforward.

With no disrespect intended to those in the prostate cancer survival world, in my experience, at least, "favorable, intermediate" prostate cancer does *not* really compare with stage IV NSCLC. Rightly or wrongly, I compared my prostate cancer to something like a torn ACL that professional athletes deal with all the time: a very serious injury of sorts, but not life-threatening. It was simply a "thing." I could get the prostate snipped out and solve the problem in one (painful) fell swoop. I could go through an interesting second bout of radiation with radiation pellets implanted in that place where the sun doesn't shine. I could wait and see what developed, which, you may recall, was the advice of the well-meaning doctor who told me I was going to die of lung cancer anyway. Or I could reach into our checking account and pay for some razzle-dazzle moves.

By this point, I was feeling confident in my roles as self-doctor and citizen-scientist. I chose the outside-the-box option. This was purely strategic. The success rate for laser ablation on "favorable, intermediate" prostate cancer is pretty amazing. My body didn't need any more radiation, not if I had other choices. And surgery really seemed like taking a sledgehammer to a penny nail. Too radical and final for my tastes. I chose the equivalent of a half-day "fight," laying on my stomach, traveling back home to Kansas City the next day, and then navigating the delicate process of using a catheter for thirty to forty days. I didn't take the second cancer too seriously, and I *don't think* I felt all that sorry for myself, but others may have differing views on this.

If you happen to be one of those 8 percent who are diagnosed with a second cancer, the same *practical* issues we have been discussing apply to second cancers as well. Do not accept conventional wisdom at face value. Do your own research. Make an informed decision about what makes sense. Get a second opinion. Take your roles as self-doctor and citizen-scientist seriously. Determine whether complementary medicine is your friend. Assess which diets or supplements, if any, are in order. These are the core issues related to any second cancer. Depending on the nature of the second cancer, there may be others, including the more philosophical issues we have already discussed.

o o o

I was coasting along quite well in the summer of 2022. I had been off active conventional treatment for about a year, and I had recovered from the laser ablation procedure applied to the cancer in my prostate. Things were looking up. I had even started this book in earnest.

Was it possible that I had put two separate cancers and almost thirty months of cancer treatments in the rear-view mirror? The answer looked like a depressing no. A CT scan that summer showed a lymph node—one of the original offenders—had grown. This led to a PET scan, which showed several lymph nodes lighting up, as well as the same spot on my spine *and* a new area of concern in my left lung. The good news? The original tumor in my right lung seemed to be no more than a shell of its former self, kind of like the rusting hull of a once imposing ship. I took heart from this—the "worst offender" was still dormant and maybe even on life support. Back to the drawing board. The recurrence offered another chance to go through the paces we have been discussing. Assessment of options. A second opinion from MD Anderson in Houston on treatment options. A serious opportunity to fight and surrender simultaneously. Making full use of acupuncture and high-dose vitamin C. As you know, I ended up doing four rounds of the original chemotherapy regimen. Then I spent twenty days in radiation ablation therapy for an hour a day. This second round of radiation targeted each of the five spots that lit up on the PET scan, and I assure you its aftermath was no fun at all. Yes, trying a legal case the second time is quite unpleasant, but there aren't too many surprises in second trials. There is always the chance to do a better job, and winning a second time around is most gratifying.

In a few respects, a recurrence will present novel issues, as did mine. But in principle, the issues we have already discussed remain just as relevant and just as potent the second or third time around.

Chapter 20: *Passing It On—*
Helping Others with Cancer

As a cancer survivor, you are uniquely qualified to help cancer patients.
    —COMPASS ONCOLOGY, *Cancer Survivorship: How You Can*
    Help Others as a Cancer Survivor

WHEN I WAS FIRST GETTING RADIATION IN HOUSTON, TEXAS, IN early 2020, thousands of miles from home, I was gone from our home for three weeks. My wife came to see me on one of the weekends during that time frame. This was mid-February 2020, just as the COVID pandemic was coming to life. For context, when I arrived in Houston for radiation, there was no pandemic. By the time I left Houston three weeks later, I was barely able to get a plane flight home.

My wife, Rebecca, had left ten or twelve days earlier, mainly to get back to our daughter, Jacqulyn. On the plane flight home, she happened to be seated next to a senior executive at one of America's largest and most profitable supermarket chains. Because Rebecca is such a delightful and open person, they ended up having an amazing discussion. It turns out that this executive spoke with an impediment, the result of cancer in his mouth. The cancer was in remission at that point, but my wife's new friend mentioned that every year or two "I need to take care of that little motherfucker." During the flight, Rebecca and her new friend had a deeply meaningful conversation about cancer survival. Before the plane landed, my wife asked this wonderful man, "What is the most important advice you would give my husband at this time?" His response? First, he said I needed to get through this initial storm. Then he added, "After that, he needs to make sure to help others. That is the key. You've got to help others with cancer."

In my experience, this stranger was and is right. This is borne out by others who have survived cancer, but those in the medical community as well. In their book *Inner Fire*, the Rosenbaums refer to this activity as actively seeking for ways to help others.[109] The Rosenbaums consider this to be a 'vital' principle in cancer survival."[110] Or, as stage IV NSCLC survivor, Colleen Connel Ziegler puts it, "I've done a lot of mentoring and advocacy over the years … for fellow lung cancer patients. One thing I am sure of is the importance of hope. It is a large and important component of this disease."[111]

By now, you have undoubtedly become aware of many others diagnosed with cancer in your circle of friends and acquaintances. I highly recommend that you make yourself available for those people who come across your path. These are your chances to pass it on, to provide others with hope. I have had dozens of such meetings or conversations, and they benefited me far more, I am willing to bet, than they benefited the newly diagnosed. What is your role in such discussions or situations? Don't worry about that. Listen to your inner voice. Most importantly, listen to the person across from you and honestly answer their questions. You will know your role. There is no need for a script or an outline of duties. Nobody can help a would-be cancer survivor like another cancer survivor.

There is a strong tradition of this kind of fellowship in the "recovery" movement for those battling addiction. For instance, in the fellowship of Alcoholics Anonymous, the famous Twelve Steps are the cornerstone for those recovering from the unmanageable effects of alcohol and drugs. The twelfth step of AA states the following: "Having had a spiritual awakening as a result of these steps, we tried to carry this message to alcoholics and to practice these principles in all our affairs."[112] The lynchpin of Step Twelve is one alcoholic in recovery helping another alcoholic. The cofounder of AA, Bill W., describes the effect of this brand of fellowship in this way: "You can help when no one else can. You can secure their confidence when others fail. Remember they are very ill."[113]

o o o

A sober person in AA is said to be either recovered or "in recovery." In the literature on cancer, there is also much that is accurately said about "recovering" from cancer. Applying the term recovery in the context of Phases Two, Three and Four, "passing it on" is, in and of itself, a parallel treatment silo that will not only help another cancer patient newly in your shoes but will also help *your* recovery. In Part Four, we see this in the stories of advanced lung cancer survivors time and again.

The lesson here?

Do *yourself* a favor, and others too: make it a point to help your comrades diagnosed with cancer. Pass it on.

Chapter 21: *Adjusting Your Visualizations*

I'm going to give you a little advice. ... All you have to do is ... stop thinking, let things happen, and be the ball.

—TY WEBB, *Caddyshack*

EARLIER, WE DISCUSSED YOUR INITIAL VISUALIZATIONS. I ALSO mentioned to you that six of seven of the visualizations I used in the first twelve months after diagnosis had come to pass.

In case you have been wondering, the one visualization that did *not* come to pass involved my teeing off on the first hole of an amateur national championship. I had specifically visualized this in great detail. The problem? I had waited until the very last day of the deadline to compete in a final tournament in the state of New York, and I canceled my plane flight to New York because it looked *certain* that the tournament would be rained out the next day. It turned out that they actually played the soggy tournament. But for a rash decision to avoid a useless plane flight, I would have been able to compete in the national championship and touch the base on every visualization I had formulated.

So I screwed the logistics of that visualization up, but don't count that against the power of visualization. As you progress through Phases Two and Three, there will be opportunities to adjust your visualizations. You may even find it useful to do so in light of the annual benchmarks we have been discussing. Remember, as Michael Lloyd says, "You can do it any way you want. ... There is no right or wrong here, just whatever you can make work."[114] And it is important that the visualization have emotional resonance. "The key here is that simply imagining an outcome does not appear to change much. But when we *feel* something in an embodied way, measurable change may occur."[115]

As I finish writing this book, for instance, one of my visualizations is a celebration of the five-year anniversary date of my diagnosis. This visualization involves a warm-weather climate, access to some very nice golf courses, a rented house large enough to accommodate some close family and friends, and a three-day weekend on or about January 20, 2025. I can see and smell the ocean waves right now, and by the time you read this, the plane tickets will already have been bought.

PART IV

Replenished Hope and Survivor Role Models

When life deals you the cancer card, make your own deck with special role models to help you remember how strong a person with cancer can be.

—FELICIA MITCHELL, "Remembering Cancer Role Models," *Cure Today*, August 15, 2018

A large number of studies show that having hope is very important for those who are ill. Hope makes ill people feel better, improves their mood, strengthens their motivation to undergo treatment and may even increase the chance that treatments are successful.

—BERT MUSSCHENGA, *Is There a Problem with False Hope?*

Chapter 22: *Understanding the Importance of Replenished Hope*

I have learned to embrace ... the cancer. I have become more educated, more compassionate, and more intensely alive than ever. ... I am strengthened by holding onto these stories of hope. The experience of others educates and enriches me, replenishing me so I can go forward, renewed.

—NILA W., metastatic lung cancer survivor

AS I HAVE MENTIONED, IF ONE OF THE MOST IMPORTANT ARROWS in one's quiver is the will to live, then hope can be considered that arrow's sharpener. There are different ways to use this sharpener, but one of the most powerful, in my opinion, is looking to role models who resonate with *your* survival experience. As Nila W. states above, stories of other survivors are a way of replenishing one's hope.

Like any type of energy supply, hope, indeed, must be replenished. In Phase Four, years five through ten of the NSCLC survival process, the examples of long-term survivors serve this function in two ways: first, just the stories alone replenish the fuel of hope, and second, the stories reaffirm those *strategies that work*. In my writing of this book, I have reviewed, interviewed, or researched the survival stories of well over several hundred cancer survivors of almost every kind. In each of these stories, *with only one exception*, the survivor had useful information about survival, either through words or actions.

149

The stories we are going to discuss in this part IV are the stories of some of the truly notorious ones. Each of these stories stands on its own; significantly, however, each of the stories is also quite connected, and I will indicate below how they have resonated with me. What is provided in this part of the book are seven stories of *realistic* hope. The stories are realistic because the people discussed are just like you and me, and, as such, their survival examples can be used to replenish the energy of *our* survival experience. As you read the accounts of advanced-stage lung cancer survivors, you will see several recurring themes: first, their strong will to live; second, some form of rekindling of the will to live; and third, a strong motivation to help others with cancer.

Before we hear these additional stories, however, I think it important to address an issue that sometimes comes up, usually from persons of a, *ahem*, self-proclaimed *scientific* mindset: Do the stories of long-term survivors provide the rest of us with "false hope"?

Chapter 23: *Rejecting the Notion of "False Hope"*

It's simple: These people who traffic in this false hope business have never been told they are going to die.

—M. WARREN and T. JUNOD, "Why There is Nothing False about 'False Hope,'" *Esquire*

LET ME CUT TO THE CHASE: THERE IS NO SUCH THING AS "FALSE hope."

False hope, in this context, is a figment in the imaginations of those who have the luxury of pondering such things. Cancer survivors do not talk about false hope—others might, but in my experience, cancer *survivors* generally do not, and long-term survivors certainly do not. Because this phrase comes up occasionally, it is important to address it now as we begin to learn from and become replenished by the stories of long-term advanced lung cancer survivors.

Let's start with a hypothetical. Let's first assume you are a newly minted Phase Two NSCLC cancer survivor, well into, say, the sixth month of survival postdiagnosis. A neighbor comes by one day with a "congratulations" present for having powered through a couple of rounds of chemotherapy. The present is gift-wrapped, and as you are unwrapping it, your neighbor advises that she only has one purpose in giving you this book: "I want you to be inspired by the author who was diagnosed with stage IV NSCLC, and wrote a book about it. I hope this inspires you to keep going through your treatments." You continue to unwrap the book and find it is Sophie Sabbage's *The Cancer Whisperer*, a book I have quoted rather extensively in these pages.

Here is the question: Has your neighbor and friend given you "false hope" by gifting you this book? I am guessing you would understand that the very specific answer is obviously no. You are already a stage IV NSCLC cancer survivor. You have already learned a few things about your disease. You have already been through some treatments. You know how to filter information about your condition at this point. Whether it's your doctor or, say, your brother-in-law mentioning a risk of "false hope" in this context, you now have your sea legs and can appreciate the words of survivor Stephanee Lee on this subject: "I am not a child. ... These people going around talking about all us poor patients chasing false hope must think we're children, and can easily be misled ... Believe me, I know that I have Stage 4 metastatic disease inside of me, and I know exactly what the statistics say my chances of survival are. I don't need some self-appointed expert to tell me about that. And so anyone who goes around talking about false hope doesn't know what they are talking about."[116]

Stephanee Lee could not be more right and could not have said it any better.

But there is a more fundamental reason to reject the notion of "false hope": *there actually is no such thing*. A person either has hope, or they do not. Hope "is either realized or not realized; but it's never false."[117] The entire notion of false hope is a red herring, and it is important that you understand the reason why this is so.

The stories of other survivors, including those outlined below, *properly understood*, do not generate false hope. They simply generate hope itself and dispel false despair.

o o o

Let us return to the 2020 NSCLC Study one last time. As the authors of the 2020 NSCLC Study began their discussion of survival rates for the 2020 sample, they made an interesting and perplexing comment: "At the start of the study of the long-term survival predictors of patients with late-stage NSCLC, the researchers equipped themselves with the knowledge from studies on stages IIIB and IV patients [and which] pathological types would accurately predict prognosis. However, in stage IV with at least 3 months of survival, this was not the case. The prediction results of the baseline and therapeutic features to distinguish DOD survivors from long-term AWD survivors is *too poor* to be of clinical value and to answer in individual patients the question 'How long do I have?'"[118]

In lay terms, the authors were stumped as to why some NSCLS patients survived and others did not. Then, quite reasonably from a scientific research perspective, the researchers kicked the can down the road and stated, "the predictive value of other features and interventions discussed should be investigated in the worldwide very large group of stage IV NSCLC patients with >3 months survival."[119] More bluntly, the authors were perplexed as to why some stage IV NSCLC survivors survive beyond Phases Two, Three, or Four, and others do not.

I agree with the authors of the 2020 NSCLC Study, but if you are reading this book, there is a very strong chance that you have neither the time nor the inclination to wait for some yet-to-be-conducted worldwide study. And there is no need for a "worldwide" study: you are an n of 1; you are fully able to dig around for examples of survivors of stage IV NSCLC, advanced lung cancer, or any other kind of cancer. In fact, I am recommending that you do just that and create *your* "special deck" of survivor role models. These survivors are closer to you than you might think. These survivors are in your community, can be found on the bookshelves of new and used bookstores, and are readily accessible on internet forums related to virtually every type of cancer. In the words of Nina W. quoted above, each of us can create this special deck of role models to help us "remember how strong a person with cancer can be."

You have already heard my thoughts on the matter. Now let's hear the stories and thoughts of other long-term lung cancer survivors.

Chapter 24: *Learning the Stories of Seven Advanced Lung Cancer Survivors*

THESE STORIES ARE OFFERED IN NO PARTICULAR ORDER OF IMPORtance. I have included them here and referred to some of them already in this book because they have each inspired me over the past five years. My mix, however, is not likely to be the same as your mix. Like many of the suggestions I am making throughout these pages, it is not as important that we make the same choices about these things as it is that you consciously engage in the task at hand. The process of doing this is itself a healing strategy, and I believe you will be doing yourself a disservice if you do not add *your* mix to this mix.

Morhaf Al Achkar, MD, PhD

In December, 2016, at the age of thirty-three, Dr. Al Achkar was diagnosed with Stage IV NSCLC. Dr. Al Achkar's story resonates with me because he has thought and written deeply about the subject of cancer survival. To state the obvious, not all survivors have the expertise, the time, or the motivation to do this. I am thankful that Dr. Al Achkar has these capacities.

In 2017, Dr. Al Achkar began writing the book *Roads to Meaning and Resilience with Cancer*, which I have referred to in previous chapters, and in which he narrates both his survival story and the story of thirty-nine others with advanced lung cancers.

He specifically related these stories to the issues of "meaning" and "resilience," two of the chapters addressed in this book. Dr. Al Achkar's book is, in effect, his own "special deck" of cancer survivors, and he used his background in scientific research to interview each of those thirty-nine persons.

"The author explains that those with [metastatic NSCLC] are living for years due to recent advancements in medical treatment, which is different from the previous life expectancy of only a few months."[120] Dr. Al Achkar's interviews of other survivors "aim to identify how these individuals make meaning, build resilience, and deal with the struggle of living with metastatic cancer that is nevertheless a chronic condition."

But Dr. Al Achkar is himself also a role model for all of us, as he has now survived seven years with advanced lung cancer and has, equally important, thought deeply about the issues that confront long-term survivors. As Dr. Al Achar states on his website, "Writing my memoir [second book] was my attempt to reconstruct my narrative. I did not want to be defined as a cancer patient nor as someone living with resilience despite cancer."[121] Dr. Al Achkar defines such "resilience" as the capacity to "be able to carry on despite significant challenges." Although his compilation of survivors involves mostly those in what we are referring to as Phases One and Two of the survival phases, Dr. Al Achkar is himself a long-term Phase Four survivor, now having survived nearly eight years after his diagnosis.

I highly recommend his thoughtful book, which brims with inspiration for all of us. Dr. Al Achkar is one of the notorious ones, and his book about resilience is a book about other notorious ones.

Nadine Beech

If forced to nominate a poster child for this section of the book, I would probably nominate Nadine Beech. Nadine has survived stage IV NSCLC for over twenty-five years! I learned of Nadine through our mutual friend and acupuncturist here in Kansas City. We met several times for coffee, and she provided me with great insight and her views on the survival process.

At the age of twenty-seven, Nadine was the picture of health and a nonsmoker. A native New Zealander, in 1997, she was diagnosed with NSCLC, which was staged two years later as stage IV.

When I interviewed her for the first time in the spring of 2024, her infectious enthusiasm about survival was not only evident but very motivational as well. After exchanging pleasantries, Nadine cut to the chase: "You have to be your own advocate." She mentioned this more than once. She also discussed the importance of complementary medicine—she has consistently had acupuncture since her diagnosis—and the need to do one's own research. "It's too easy to get lazy, and let the doctors do all the work."

When I asked Nadine about the importance of the will to live and a rebellious spirit, Nadine agreed these are, in effect, significant threshold issues for survivors. As just one example of this, after her diagnosis, Nadine met with her oncology team and specifically advised them to redact any references to her having a "stage IV" condition from her medical file. Intuitively, she understood the importance of words and rejected suggestions that she had a terminal condition. To this day, she maintains the importance of recontextualizing her survivor experience as a chronic condition.

After her diagnosis, Nadine changed careers and became a personal trainer, where she helps others with their fitness goals and maintains her own fitness goals directly related to her chronic condition. This is ichigo in action. She maintains a vigorous workout routine and attempts to keep her lungs as healthy as possible. She generally avoids sugar, and she continues her acupuncture treatments on a regular basis. Nadine describes her fitness goals as "constantly working hard to be the best I can be for when my cancer-free day would come. And finally, it's here."

Nadine is also a strong proponent of seeking out second opinions. "Don't expect your treatment to be a one-stop shop! You have to work hard and it is your responsibility to find all the treatments that go hand in hand with your physician's plan." It turns out that Nadine and I shared more than an acupuncturist: Nadine and I also were treated by the very same doctors at both the University of Kansas Cancer Center and MD Anderson Cancer Center.

Michael Lloyd

You have already heard from Michael Lloyd throughout this book. Michael is an example of someone who sought to deeply understand the challenges specific to the lung cancer survival process and "what it takes to beat the odds." His book *Beating Crazy Odds* is filled with specific exercises and techniques to promote healing and reverse side effects by taking a proactive approach to help restore your mind, body, and spirit to "an optimum state of health."

Michael Lloyd was diagnosed in January of 2001. "The diagnosis was an advanced case of small cell lung cancer (the fast-moving kind) with a large inoperable tumor in [his] lung that was wrapped around [his] pulmonary artery and another tumor that was located in [his] brain." In the book, Michael places major significance on "maintaining a positive winning attitude and why it is essential to surviving lung cancer." He further states, "You must truly want to survive and be willing to do whatever it takes to overcome anything and everything that gets in the way. That's the attitude you need, first and foremost, to succeed."[122] He also discusses the importance of breathing and visualization techniques.

Here is how Michael sums up the major lessons of his advanced lung cancer survival: "Somewhere between maintaining a positive attitude, being actively engaged in the decisions I faced, minimizing stress, eating well, breathing and visualization techniques, loving, laughing, prayer and forgiveness, in conjunction with conventional treatments; I created a magical combination with help and guidance from the outside and orchestrated from within that brought me back to an optimum state of health."[123]

Michael is also a strong advocate of meeting with and helping others with cancer: "I cannot begin to express the look in their eyes as they hung on every word. They were starving for direction and extremely grateful to receive advice from a survivor."[124]

Published in 2014, Michael's book and related website is a very nuts-and-bolts summary of some specific steps he undertook to become a long-term lung cancer survivor. The book is a very straightforward approach to lung cancer and is, in my opinion, an excellent starting point for those recently diagnosed with any form of cancer, let alone advanced lung cancer.

Richard Bloch

Some survivors will resonate with you because of their personal example of breaking through the difficulties inherent in survival. Others will resonate with you because of their written words. Others will resonate because of their actions in helping others and their advocacy on behalf of others with cancer. Richard Bloch resonates with me for all of these reasons.

Richard Bloch was the cofounder and honorary chairman of the Board of H&R Block, Inc., the tax advisory firm that many of us have heard of over the past few decades. As you know, both he and his wife, Annette, have written extensively about surviving and fighting cancer. They also have put significant money behind those words, including substantial funding for the cancer center where I have received most of my treatments.

Richard Bloch was diagnosed with what was considered "terminal" cancer in 1978 and given three months to live. He died of a heart condition twenty-six years later in 2004.

In my mind, Richard Bloch was and is the true embodiment of a long-term cancer survivor. He and his wife Annette devoted their lives to improving the lives of others who are diagnosed with cancer by founding the RA Bloch Cancer Foundation in 1980. Always positive, they educated and motivated people to "fight to live and beat their disease." The books written by the Blochs, although written almost forty years ago, still possess state-of-the-art advice for surviving *any* type of cancer. To reiterate some of those words: "The biggest and hardest single thing that you will be required to do in the entire battle is to make up your mind to really fight ... You must, on your own, make the commitment that you will do everything in your power to fight your disease."[125]

The Blochs epitomize the "pass-it-on" mentality. As I have mentioned, the Blochs have also underwritten cancer survivor parks throughout the country with inspiring quotes and sculptures for the general public. These parks are refuges within a number of metropolitan areas solely dedicated to cancer survival. I am blessed that one such park is less than a half-mile from our house in Kansas City. I was walking through that park one day, during the writing of this book, and came across a placard with a quote on it under the capitalized word COMMITMENT: "The biggest and the hardest single thing you will be required to do in the entire battle is to make up your mind to really fight it. You must, on your own, make the commitment that you will do everything in your power to fight your disease. No exceptions. Nothing halfway.

Nothing for the sake of ease or convenience. Everything! Nothing short of it. When you have done this, you have accomplished the most difficult thing you will have to accomplish throughout your entire treatment."

Nothing halfway. Nothing for the sake of ease or convenience. It is important that you savor these words. These words are the will to live in action.

Rick Fields

Rick is the long-term survivor of metastatic lung cancer featured in the book *Inner Fire: Your Will to Live: Stories of Courage, Hope, and Determination*. This book was written by Ernest and Isadora Rosenbaum, authors whom I have quoted extensively throughout this book. Rick is featured in detail in chapter 9 of the Rosenbaums' book. I have never met Rick Fields in person, but you have met him in the pages of this book. Rick has been a survivor story I have shared with others in the drafts of this book and in conversation. Several people I have shared Rick's story with have resonated with the term "warrior energy," a two-word summary of the mentality so crucial after a stage IV cancer diagnosis. Rick Fields is a prime example of several of the concepts we discussed in this book. I have already quoted him in a previous chapter, but his precise words in response to the grim prognosis given when diagnosed are worth repeating: "Basically, my response to my cancer always is, I'm going to live until I die. ... I told one of my doctors, 'You are also going to live until you die. You think that you know when I'm going to die. You don't even know when you yourself are going to die."[126] This is exactly the first act of rebellion we have already discussed. "My first response was definitely a warrior energy towards this cancer which I felt I had to fight."[127]

Rick is also an example of the importance of the language we use in discussing our cancer condition. When I first read about Rick's survival story, I saw someone who intuitively understood the importance of flipping conventional wisdom on its head. Amazingly, he learned this from one of his doctors. After receiving a second opinion after his initial diagnosis, a young doctor at Stanford emphasized to Rick that "incurable" does not mean *terminal*: "He told me, 'Everybody says this is incurable. ... Has anybody said to you that *incurable* does not necessarily mean terminal?'"[128]

It sounds like Rick was blessed to have a Stanford doctor who possessed some of that warrior energy too.

Jennifer Olson

Nadine Beach introduced me to Jennifer Olson, a fellow Kansas City area resident, again demonstrating that survivor role models are truly in our midst and sometimes live only a mile or two away from us.

Jennifer was diagnosed with stage IV NSCLC in April 2015. A former high school teacher in the Kansas City area at the time, she soon thereafter dedicated herself to survival by caring for her husband and three terrific children and "managing [her] chronic illness."[129] Since April of 2015, she has lived with metastatic lung cancer. Or, as she explains it more precisely, "I am living as fully as possible within the limitations of lung cancer."[130]

I interviewed Jennifer for this book in May of 2024. The wisdom and life lessons Jennifer has gained through nine-plus years of various difficult treatments and her survival story as a whole are an inspiration to any cancer patient dealing with any type of cancer. Like many of the survivors I have met, Jennifer is a student of the survival game, and she has pursued many of the strategies we have discussed throughout these pages.

Jennifer is a prime example of the importance of self-advocacy, i.e., taking responsibility for her healing. For instance, in light of her father's past health experience, postdiagnosis, Jennifer immediately understood the importance of utilizing palliative care while undergoing her standard treatments of chemotherapy and radiation. "The first step in receiving palliative care is to acknowledge that you have a chronic disease that is impacting your ability to live fully. It does not mean you are 'dying.'"[131] Jennifer is a strong advocate of this service, and, using the framework we have discussed herein, considers palliative care a significant "parallel silo" for healing and survival.

Jennifer is a role model who demonstrates the importance of passing it on. In the past decade, she and her family have focused on "raising awareness about lung cancer and staying as healthy as possible." She states, "I believe my job right now is to stay as positive as I can to further the healthiest lifestyle I can to remain cancer stable so that research can catch up and run ahead and find a cure."[132]

Having survived several rounds of chemotherapy and radiation and having endured the challenges of a recurrence, Jennifer is a long-term survivor, has lived to tell the tale, and helps others live to tell the tale. Jennifer's faith has also been important, and in our interview, she affirmed the importance of the will to live. "An important key to survival is to combine self-advocacy with all of your team (professionals to friends), treatments, faith and hope with a knowing that life is more than having a heartbeat."

Jennifer's attitude postdiagnosis was, "Yes, this sucks, and I'm still going to read my child his bedtime stories."[133] One of those children, by the way, just graduated from college in the spring of 2024.

Amanda Nerstad

I learned about Amanda Nerstad by researching the lung cancer survivor stories of others on one of the numerous lung cancer websites devoted to lung cancer. Amanda's story is publicly available online, as are many other such survivor stories, just a click away from us. In fact, there are hundreds of such stories available to you for your research in creating a "special deck" of survivors. Amanda's story resonates with me because this complete stranger—to me at least—reached many of the same conclusions about cancer survival we have been discussing in this book.

Amanda is a never-smoker who was diagnosed in 2016 with stage IV NSCLC. She was thirty-nine years old. Her doctors gave her between two weeks and nine months to live. She has now survived seven years past her diagnosis. In the wake of her diagnosis, Amanda tested positive for a mutation in the anaplastic lymphoma kinase gene, or ALK gene This mutation is found in about four percent of all cases of NSCLC.

Amanda's advice to those recently diagnosed? "1. Don't give up. ... 2. Lean on your family and support team. ... 3. Always try to find something to celebrate. ... 4. Try to do your own research. Be your own advocate. Find the best doctors for your specific cancer, seek out a second opinion. ... 5. Find a support group online for your type of cancer. ... You need just as much mental support as medicine!"[134]

Throughout her survival, Amanda has resisted the victim label and has learned to lean on her faith: "Throughout this crazy journey, it's been helpful to stay positive, thank God for our blessings, continue to make family memories and not sweat the small stuff. It's okay to have a moment. My days are not always great. If I have a bad day, I give myself 24 hours to be sad letting my mind 'go there.'"[135]Amanda is also on a mission to "spread the word about lung cancer and the importance of biomarker testing,"[136] and she and her husband Gary have taken this involvement with helping others "to the next level, fundraising for research and the ultimate goal of a cure. [Their group] has raised more than $7 million for research into ALK-positive lung cancer."[137] Amanda (and her husband, Gary) are tried-and-true examples of what it means to pass it on.

Finally, Amanda is an example of the importance of that word we've been using quite a lot in these pages. In this context, Amanda's doctor at MD Anderson after her diagnosis is especially significant: "The first thing he told us was not to give up hope. He said his job was to keep me alive until a cure was found and to stay strong and keep fighting."[138]

PART V
Rekindling Hope—Every Day, In Every Way

Survivors develop a mantra. It can be anything.
—LAURENCE GONZALES, *Deep Survival*

Coué's efforts were directed at achieving command over oneself; arousing the will to live, increasing self-responsibility ... increasing proactive initiative ... activating healing processes, arousing latent neurochemical and neurobiological resources ... promoting natural self-regulation ... strengthening the "will to health"' ... and, overall, ego-strengthening.
—YEATES, "ÉMILE Coué and His Method"

Chapter 25: *Understanding the Importance of Rekindling Hope*

The ECM is a method which everyone should follow—the sick to obtain healing, the healthy to prevent the coming of disease in the future. By its practice one can insure for ourselves, all our lives long, an excellent state of health, both of mind and body.

> ÉMILE COUÉ, from the foreword of
> *The Practice of Autosuggestion*

HOPE IS THE FUEL FOR THAT ENERGY WE ARE CALLING THE WILL to live.

But how does one *arouse* that energy over the long haul to rekindle the will to live? In other words, is there a simple and appropriate daily strategy for maintaining hope, and thus the will to live?

What if I told you that hope could be rekindled every single day before and after a stage IV NSCLC diagnosis and that the process of rekindling hope can be treated like the development of any habit—a habit that takes less than five minutes per day? Let's talk about this strategy, a strategy you can adopt *today*.

As we have discussed, the method of rekindling hope that I have employed is the method of Émile Coué. The ECM is, in the words of one expert, a particular strategy for "achieving command over oneself [and] arousing the will to live."[139] More specifically, the ECM is a twice-daily practice of arousing and thus rekindling the will to live. Stripped of its theoretical framework and doctrinal underpinnings, the ECM is the equivalent of a twice-daily exercise routine for the person who might be training for a marathon or a tennis tournament. And, like any exercise routine, momentum begets momentum (i.e., the more one engages the ECM, the more second nature the method becomes).

Before we discuss more of the particulars of the ECM, let's first explore the psychological technique that drives the ECM. That technique is called autosuggestion.

Chapter 26: *Incorporating Autosuggestion into Your Healing*

Most mental processes occur outside our conscious awareness and beyond our control.

—YEATES, "ÉMILE Coué and His Method," Section II, 8

AS I MENTION IN THE "BEGINNINGS" SECTION OF THIS BOOK, SINCE mid-January of 2020, I have recited, "Every day, in every way, I am getting better and better," twenty times in the morning and twenty times in the evening, every single day, with only a handful of exceptions. I have endeavored to recite these lines in the morning while coming out of sleep and in the evening while drifting off into sleep.

Forty times per day, approximately fifteen hundred-plus days. I have recited this simple mantra over seventy thousand times. If it is true that, as Gonzales says, "survivors develop a mantra," this has been my mantra for roughly five years.

I am of two minds about this chapter. In an earlier draft, this chapter was going to be a *primary* focus of the book. Later on, I thought this section might be best left out of the book. For context, I have shared some versions of this chapter with a fair number of close friends and other acquaintances with a recent cancer diagnosis. The feedback in response to this chapter has been a mixed bag of polite silence and muted enthusiasm. For example, I shared this chapter with a very successful doctor in my community, a doctor diagnosed with a form of stage IV cancer, and he has more or less not spoken to me since.

Some of these reactions have led me to be reticent about adding this section, but I have erred on the side of including this information. Ultimately, the decision was this simple: what follows in this section actually happened to me, and I consider my deployment of this particular daily habit to surviving cancer to have been a substantial factor in my cancer survival. Because my narrated events about the use of the ECM are *true*, I have concluded that they *may* be useful to you in your survival, your sense of peace, and in the rekindling of hope, and thus, your will to live. Your mileage may vary, as the kids sometimes say.

Let's first cover some background. I have been a lifelong student of the "mental game" associated with a number of activities, such as trial lawyering, golf, and martial arts. The mental game is, for our purposes, the development of the *skill* of using one's subconscious mind to assist in the performance of seemingly conscious tasks. The term "mental game" was actually coined by a tennis pro, Timothy Gallwey, in the 1970s, who quite accidentally learned that his tennis students performed better when they took their active consciousness in the performance of physical tasks, such as the execution of a serve.[140]

Before I was diagnosed with cancer, in my office, that for a short time became a War Room and then became the Peace Room, one bookshelf contained at least twenty volumes dealing with one or another facet of the mental game. The subjects range from tennis and golf to martial arts and trial lawyering. There were and still are several additional volumes on the workings of the subconscious mind, consistent with the mental-game genre of books. Thus, quite by happenstance, prior to my diagnosis, I had been a student of the mental-game literature for at least twenty years. And, equally important, I had *applied* the mental-game concepts to golf, martial arts, and my occupation as a trial lawyer.

During my crash course on cancer in the wake of the diagnosis I have already described, I was very surprised to see that nobody seemed to have written extensively on the mental game of cancer, nor were there many articles directly on point. It seemed quite intuitive to me, even at that very early stage, that whatever the doctors decided was necessary, there would be no question but that I would need to add my own efforts at healing. I just couldn't easily find anything that hit the mark. How could there be a book about the healing power of carrot juice and sauerkraut but *not* a book about the mental game of cancer? Very strange.

Then I learned about an interesting Frenchman who lived in the last half of the nineteenth century by the name of Émile Coué. Coué was something of a chemist and a hypnotist in the late 1800s. He dispensed "medicinal remedies" to his patients on a daily basis. After some time, he observed that when he encouraged his patients that they would improve with the taking of the medicine, those patients *markedly* improved. In other words, his mere *suggestion* that they would improve enhanced the efficacy of the treatment. This observation was the genesis of his development of the ECM.

Eventually, Coué wrote a book about the power of such suggestion and more or less invented a way for his patients *themselves* to implant such suggestions. Coué termed this technique "auto-suggestion." His particular form of suggestion, a mantra of sorts—"Every day, in every way, I am getting better and better"— is a very simple form of autosuggestion. Coué observed that such autosuggestion was most efficacious when repeated around twenty times in the morning and twenty times at night, in the "between" state of sleep and waking, and then waking and sleep, otherwise known as the hypnagogic state.

At the turn of the twentieth century, Coué became world famous for the healings that occurred when his patients adopted this method. He traveled the world and lectured on the everyday way of self-healing he called autosuggestion. The Beatles even made a song about this mantra.

As I read more about Coué and some other authors who had expounded on the theories of autosuggestion in early 2020, I saw no reason *not* to adopt his proposed mantra and have been using it ever since.

o o o

The power of the ECM requires a thorough understanding of the power of suggestion, so let's begin this discussion of suggestion with a hypothetical: Assume you have been driving on a highway and, quite suddenly, are rear-ended by a semitruck. Before losing consciousness, the last thing you remember is a final glance in the rearview mirror, and the image of a large truck approaching. You wake up some unknown time later, pulled from your car, strapped in the back of an ambulance, and a paramedic, reading from a script unbeknownst to you, suggests to you the following:

> *The worst is over. We are taking you to the hospital.*
> *Everything is being made ready. Let your body concentrate*
> *on repairing itself and feeling secure. ... Things are being*
> *made ready at the hospital for you. We're getting there as*
> *quickly and safely as possible. You are now in a safe position.*
> *The worst is over.*[141]

> —Donald Trent Jacobs, Patient Communication
> for First Responders and EMS Personnel

In the above hypothetical, the paramedic is engaging in what is called "suggestion"—she is communicating to you the *suggestion*, in less than thirty seconds, that things are only going to *get better* ("the worst is over."). The paramedic is doing so while you are in something of an altered or trance state—the state of having just regained consciousness after a traumatic accident.

What might be the effect of such suggestions? Interestingly, this exact suggestion was the basis of a remarkable study of how very simple communicational elements, made in an optimal way under specific circumstances, can make medical treatment more effective.[142] The study sought to compare "typical" accident victims with a suggestion control group in which the above-quoted script was given to injured accident victims. One group was treated in a random, haphazard fashion—as are most accident victims—and the other was specifically provided the above assurances by an authority figure (the paramedic), in the form of suggestion. The results of the suggestion on the control group were marked: "The half-minute intervention resulted in an increased survival rate during transport to the hospital, shorter hospital stays, and faster recovery in the members of the suggestion group."[143]

Common sense tells us the power of suggestion is obviously not limited to paramedics, and various scientific studies have demonstrated this in other contexts. Other examples of this same principle in the scientific literature involve the use of suggestion via a twelve-minute taped message to anesthetized patients, the use of suggestion to a comatose patient to increase their chance of survival, and the inducement of speedier recoveries by a practitioner's simple and basic description of the proper functioning of the immune system.[144]

Researcher Katalin Varga describes the power of suggestion in this way. "It has been clear for hundreds of years: words have power." This is especially true in the medical setting. Thus, "all the elements of medical communications—e.g., introducing our clinic on the website, decorating our waiting room, reporting the diagnosis, explaining the planned intervention, telling the prognosis or death of a relative, just to mention a few—may have a suggestive effect even if we know nothing about the suggestive method."[145]

Varga's focus in the above research relates primarily to third-party suggestion, but the ECM is a form of autosuggestion. In my view, autosuggestion—self-directed suggestion—is more applicable to persons with long-term diseases. Rather than being guided by an *outside* party, the subject—in our case, the person with cancer—guides himself in terms of thoughts, feelings, or beliefs.

According to Coué's contemporary C. Harry Brooks, the process of autosuggestion consists of two steps. The first step is the acceptance of an idea. The second step is the transformation of that idea into reality:

Both these operations are performed by the Unconscious. Whether the idea originated in the mind of the subject or is presented without by the agency of another person is a matter of *indifference. In both cases it undergoes the same process. It is submitted to the Unconscious, accepted or rejected, and so either realized or ignored. ...* In essentials all suggestion is Autosuggestion. *The only distinction ... is between spontaneous Autosuggestion,* which takes place independently of our will and choice, *and induced Autosuggestion, in which* we consciously select the ideas we wish to realize and purposely convey them to the Unconscious.[146] (Emphasis added.)

In the above quote, Brooks uses the term *Unconscious* for the term *subconscious* we have used so far in this book. If we harken back to our hypothetical paramedic scenario, the idea that "the worst is over" was suggested to the accident victim, and then the accident victim's body, via the subconscious, was thus provided an anchored suggestion for transforming that idea into reality.

The question then becomes: Can one get the same benefits of suggestion by, in effect, eliminating the middleman, or third party?

The answer, according to Coué, is yes. You, the cancer survivor, can take advantage of these principles of autosuggestion on a twice-daily basis. The ECM thereby becomes a simple, elegant technique for supercharging your body in the service of healing by intentionally using your subconscious mind and your imagination in the service of healing. I am not aware of any author or doctor who has tied the ECM, or anything like the ECM, to the rekindling of the will to live. But, as we now know, the issue of hope is integral to the will to live, and the ECM is nothing if not a daily reminder of hope: *Every day, in every way, I'm getting better and better.* What could be more hopeful than this?

The "magic" of the ECM is that the mantra works on two separate fronts. One must be conscious enough to remember to do the mantra. One must *also* be unconscious enough—in the state between sleep and wakefulness—for the anchoring of hope to occur. Have I "scientifically" tested this? No. But I am an "n of 1," just like you, and I can think of no valid reason a person attempting to survive cancer would *not* engage the ECM as a parallel silo of healing in all Phases of survival.

o o o

There is a respectable intellectual tradition to support the use of something like the ECM. Aristotle, one of the great Greek sages, a scientific genius, and perhaps the father of Western philosophy, famously said, "A vivid imagination compels the body to obey it." Taken literally, Aristotle's insight is that the human mind can—via a vivid imagination—*modify the body*. Ralph Waldo Emerson, the famed Transcendentalist philosopher and American sage of the nineteenth century, said, "What lies behind us and what lies before us are tiny matters compared to what lies within us." Taken literally, Emerson's insight was that an actual, present power—something which lies within us—can overcome the past and shape outcomes in the future. Emerson implied that this internal hinge was far *greater* than we understood. And, especially in this context, the well-known words of Albert Einstein are worth quoting as well: "Imagination is more important than knowledge. Knowledge is limited. Imagination encircles the world." The list of quotes from various sages from virtually every era and intellectual tradition could go on and on.

Coué took the insights of sages such as Aristotle, Emerson, and Einstein quite literally. Fortunately for those Coué treated, his curiosity led to the development of an original approach to healing that was entirely within the control of the *patient*, the person who suffered from the ailment in need of healing. Fortunately for those like me and others with health problems, both major and minor, Coué translated these insights into a practice that is available to literally anybody, easy to understand, and quite simple to execute.

Perhaps most fortunate of all, the ECM costs nothing, is a parallel treatment silo that does not contradict any medical treatment modality and is entirely within the cancer survivor's control to execute. In other words, the ECM is *freely* available, freely understandable, and free.

The ECM—although more than a hundred years old—is a surprisingly cutting-edge technique for rekindling hope and healing from disease.

o o o

If you have read this far, you understand the gist of the ECM. Before reading any further, please sit down and try the ECM. Relax your mind a little bit and say to yourself, "Every day, in every way, I am getting better and better." Then, repeat this nineteen more times. The ECM calls for you to do this again tonight before you go to sleep. If there is a noisy voice in your head offering resistance to this experiment, ignore that voice.

What do you have to lose?

Chapter 27: *Applying the Method of Émile Coué Daily*

By the use of this method each of us should be able to look forward to a life in which disease is a diminishing factor. But how great a part it will play depends on the conditions we start from and the regularity and correctness of our practice. Should disease befall us we possess within a potent means of expelling it, but this does not invalidate destroying it from without. Autosuggestion and the usual medical practice go hand in hand, each supplementing each other.

—C. HARRY Brooks, 111–112

THE ECM IS THE SPECIFIC STRATEGY TO REKINDLE, ON A REGULAR basis, one's personal hope for surviving cancer.

I do not claim that is the only way to do this. There may be other, more forceful ways to rekindle hope and, thus, the will to live, such as prayer, meditation, or even exercise. It is only in hindsight that I have seen how, *for me*, the ECM has sharpened that arrow in the quiver we have been calling the will to live. And, for what it is worth, I truly do not believe I would be alive today were it not for my having stumbled across the power of autosuggestion embodied in the ECM. The beauty of the ECM is that it works hand-in-glove with all of the other strategies we have discussed in this book, including traditional cancer treatments. The convenience of the ECM is that you need not wait to begin the method. The power of the ECM is that it is a daily practice, and thus a daily reminder, of the need and capacity to arouse one's will to live.

I hope you have been convinced to give the ECM serious attention in aid of your survival from advanced lung cancer (or any other health challenge). If the ECM is not your cup of tea, use your role as a self-doctor and citizen-scientist to explore other daily practices that might resonate more forcefully with your path of cancer survival.

Whether you adopt the ECM or something else, please remember there is a mental side to surviving cancer. Those who do not employ this mental game on a regular basis are fighting cancer with one hand tied behind their back.

CONCLUSION

What you have read in this book is probably different from anything you have ever quite believed about your body and its functions. My hope is that, at some level at least, parts of it make some sense to you... Only after you have tried something, do you have the right to say with authority that it is not for you.

—RICHARD AND ANNETTE BLOCH, *Fighting Cancer*

IT IS AN UNFORTUNATE FACT THAT MANY WHO ARE DIAGNOSED with stage IV lung cancer do not survive long enough to write or think deeply about the process of cancer survival. This unfortunate fact leads to yet another strange paradox: those who *do* survive long enough to write about the survival process can be tempted to believe they are unique, lucky, or possess special insights about survival. I claim none of these things and hope *you* now understand that *you* need not be unique, lucky, or have special insights to survive. I hope you now understand that what is urgently required is a passionate will to live and a conscious strategy for strengthening, nourishing, and cultivating that will to live. This will not *ensure* your survival, but it may, if given due attention and regard, maximize your *chances* of survival. Attention and regard for one's will to live can then become a habit, and that habit will become a driving force in your life.

o o o

I was having lunch with a long-time friend a few months ago as I was completing a draft of this book. The topic of the role of the will to live came up. My friend John, a trial lawyer, very understandably asked, "Are you saying that someone with cancer riddling his entire body can survive a serious cancer by simply having a 'will to live'?"

I thought about the question for a moment and stalled a little bit by telling him that he was asking a very good question. I harkened back to that gray afternoon from over four years ago, the afternoon my wife, Rebecca, gave me "the talk." Then I responded, "The 'will to live' is an energetic capacity. The fact that this energy is not much talked about or well understood in the context of cancer survival does not mean it is a 'miracle cure' or anything like that. I believe that the will to live is simply an independent strategy related to healing, but it must be consciously employed. I know this because I have felt this in my life. It has helped me survive far longer than I was supposed to."

I then added, "The 'will to live' doesn't trump medical treatments. What the 'will to live' does is add a mental-game element to healing. Harnessing the 'will to live' makes such treatments more effective. This is the lesson of survivors in almost every survival setting, not just cancer."

John was warming up to what I was saying, but he still seemed less than fully convinced. I then looked at him very directly, just as I would you, the reader, if the two of us were having lunch right now. I concluded, "There is no reason for someone fighting cancer not to do this. They need to *use* this arrow on purpose, but the arrow can dull sometimes. It needs to be sharpened." Now John seemed convinced.

∘ ∘ ∘

My hope is that you are convinced as well. Remember: no matter which phase of cancer survival you are in right now, your situation is still very grave.

I wish you the best—every day, in every way.

Afterword

BY REBECCA BOGGS SEYFERTH, PHD

I HAVE LIVED THROUGH AND AM A WITNESS TO ALL THAT IS WRITten herein. My heart lived it, my soul lived it, and my body took on the burden, heaviness, and grief that stage IV lung cancer introduces to a family.

My body did not experience getting a port surgically inserted. My body did not feel the effects of chemotherapy coursing through the system of blood, cells, and veins; nor did it feel the utter depletion and exhaustion of the entire physical/organic enterprise after a course of radiation. As the caregiver, I was pummeled in a different way. I grieved and mourned the loss of life as it was "BC," before cancer—life as it was when a steady paycheck was taken for granted; life as it was before the gut-wrenching diet of yo-yo emotions; life as it was when it was possible to plan one's schedule a month or two in advance.

Like all caregivers, I grieved never being able to feel "normal" while tending to my husband and witnessing him suffer. I yearned for the life rhythm of semipredictability, as my innards were in near constant turmoil. I lamented my current state of living and the palpable uncertainty of how this long-haul cancer battle would end. Without a doubt, caregivers walk through their own Valley of the Shadow of Death. Alongside their suffering beloved, they also dwell in a world of surreal death-in-life, and are disturbingly separated from the normal flow of the healthy world. Mistress Mayhem who, with great cruelty, toys with one's heart, gut, and emotions, most certainly visits *both* patient and caregiver. One can move from the lowest pit of despair to the highest mountain of hope within the span of a day, an hour, or even a minute. Needless to say, experiencing such extreme vacillations of mind wreaks havoc on the entirety of one's being. Perhaps you can identify with some of this experience.

Now, let me tell you about something so surprisingly amazing that happened either despite or because of all this: Five years after his initial diagnosis, Paul and I are both better humans. Our lives are simply better, every day and in every way.

In the preface of this book, Paul tells the story of how I admonished him (when he was tempted to lull gently through death's door) not to go into that Good Night. Paul heard me loud and clear and obeyed my command.

Now let me tell you about how Paul set me straight—even before the scene that he describes. It begins with the initial discovery of the tumor on his lung.

On a freezing and inhospitable January day in 2020, Paul and I found out that the terrible cough and double pneumonia that he had been experiencing for over two months, which had been treated with continuous courses of antibiotics to no avail, was either stage III or stage IV lung cancer. We knew that something was off by the way in which the pulmonologist both entered and exited the room that day. Alarmingly, he conveyed to us "the entire story" in his first few steps. We were standing up, eager for some explanation as to why Paul's stubborn pneumonia would not go away. With scan results in hand, this doctor looked down at the floor. It was strange that he was not looking us in the eye.

Now, before I continue, it must be emphasized that this doctor was clearly a capable physician, but perhaps was accustomed to treating more run-of-the-mill maladies. But this is also true: as a human being, capable of error, he had been misdiagnosing Paul throughout his visits prior to the meeting I am describing. So, please understand that it is not my intention to entirely diminish a doctor's role in healing. Without the oncologists at MD Anderson and Kansas University Cancer Center and the traditional cancer treatments they initially prescribed, Paul most likely would not be here. What I *am* illustrating and emphasizing, however, is that doctors do not have complete power over every aspect of your inner self, your life, or your healing potential. With this caveat established, I shall continue.

Following this initial salutation of bad tidings, the doctor's scuffling and defeated body language conveyed to us something like the following:

> *The news is so awful and horrible that I need to keep looking down at the floor. This news scares even me. I am a bit ashamed and embarrassed that I have been treating you for many weeks now for something else, and these weeks were precious time that you could have been in cancer treatment. I missed it. I didn't even think about getting you a scan until it was too late. Not only do you have cancer, but it has metastasized.*

Somewhere during the beginning of this awkward interaction, the doctor told Paul that he had cancer. Pressed to escape the room, having just verbally dropped the C word on us—that anvil-like crusher hearts and perceptions—the doctor turned to leave, and yet, he had equipped us with nothing: not a tiny morsel of hope, no referrals, no advice, and, certainly, no sympathy. The doctor left us with his own sense of urgency to abruptly hightail it out of there, as he seemed to want nothing to do with helping us absorb the shock from his message of doom, so palpably felt. To release himself from this uncomfortable situation seemed to be his primary aim, but my husband detained him by making the following inquiry: "My clients, before going to trial, ask me, 'How good are my chances at winning this case?' I'm now asking you how are my chances?" The doctor's shrugged shoulders told us the answer, and he then relayed to us that there was a 95 percent chance the cancer was either stage III or stage IV.

"Do I need a cancer doctor?" Paul asked in the direction of the doctor's back as he was walking out the door. Over his shoulder, he replied, "Yes, I'll get you a referral." The door shut, and the doctor was finally free from the patient who he had treated as though he were a sort of dead man walking.

This was our first foray into the cancer world. This was also our first insult. There would be more, and you have already read about some of them in this book.

Continuing to describe the aftermath of this initial appointment is important, as it was from this point that Paul and I were to find deep, true, and practical hope. Having noted this, I will continue to tell the tale of how Paul set me right in my thinking as patient to caregiver even before we entered intensely into the world of cancer treatments.

o o o

The initial appointment with the doctor that I have described, if you recall, was in early January of 2020. Paul and I felt the bitter cold wind biting our hands and faces as we walked from the doctor's building to our car. Once protected from the elements inside the car, we spent a long period of time dazed, stunned, crushed and heartbroken, just sitting on the cold leather seats in our parkas. We stared blankly out of the frosted windshield at the dismal, hostile gusts of snow. We both cried.

Paul was in the driver's seat, I was in the passenger seat, and we held each other's bare hands tightly over the console. Through this haze of anguish, we reminded each other of how much we loved one other. Our spoken and unspoken words also conveyed something like "it has been nice" ("it" being our relationship of twenty-nine years). Our intense grieving had begun.

We had been "white-coat-pilled."

This term occurred to me just a few days ago when looking back on this crucial span of time. It is akin to being blue- or red-pilled in the modern American vernacular, only I am applying our "drinking the Kool-Aid" to how Paul and I had immediately swallowed, ingested, and absorbed this initial doctor's message without pushback, without question, and without analysis. We assumed that what the doctor said (and didn't say) was the Truth with a capital T. Period. We believed, together in the car, that our fate was sealed.

And then when Paul and I got home, Paul immediately got to work. He started to learn about the deadly disease with which he had just been diagnosed.

o o o

So, how did it then come to pass that nearly five years later, my husband is now sitting across from me in our family room as I write this, fully healthy, albeit living with disease, and feeling great, telling me his corny jokes that I still, unbelievably, find funny? He sits in his big leather chair, one of the first pieces of furniture that we had purchased in the early days of marriage. He sits in it like King Paul, watching a Kansas City Royals game on his iPad, having just put down a book (and before that, having purchased, hauled in, and put away a full load of groceries!). From where we were five years ago, many voices would say that this is too good to be true. But it is true. It is real. I see it, I am living it, and I am witnessing it firsthand.

How did it come to pass that Paul would survive two bouts of chemotherapy and two rounds of high dose radiation, survive an additional cancer, and write the book you now have in hand? How did he endure the unavoidable pain of the healing treatments—the bouts of nausea, the experience of metal mouth, the neuropathy, the ruthless exhaustion, and the visits to emergency rooms?

Here is my way of answering this question.

Early on, Paul had to *decide who* he is and *whose* he is. Did the essence of his being solely belong to the doctors? Did he have agency to steer his own ship in ways that were in his control, and if so, to what extent? The deeper question was and still remains: What is it, beyond the physical, that can broaden and magnify a patient's vision (or anyone's for that matter) so that one can truly *see, taste,* and *feel* the possibility of healing from a deadly disease? Here, a refresher of two relevant quotes from Paul's book are most salient: Albert Einstein: "Imagination is more important than knowledge: Knowledge is limited; imagination encircles the world." And then Aristotle: "A vivid imagination compels the body to obey it."

So, here is the question: *Who* are you and *whose* are you?

In Mary Shelley's famous novel of 1818, *Frankenstein,* the doctor creates life from death through tissue, veins, skin and electric shock. Shelley's novel poses the questions "What is life? What creates life? What animates us?" Are we not more than mere electric impulses and sinews, blood and bone?

Dr. Frankenstein does not understand the complexity of the Creature that he pieced together, who has feelings, yearnings, and desires. Like any patient or any human, the Creature craves companionship, kindness, and sympathy. The doctor is horrified and appalled that this living thing not only has blood that courses through his veins, and a heart that pumps it, but also a will to live that embraces fully deeper human qualities of love, comfort, and belonging.

This may seem irrelevant to my husband's book and your very grave situation, but I assure you it is quite relevant.

Paul Seyferth *decided* that there was more to him and more to his healing than what the doctors saw. Of course, we needed the expertise and guidance of those who wear the white coats. But there was so much more.

Love is powerful medicine.

If you are alone, learn to love your being and the essence of who you are.

If you are blessed to have loving caregivers, use that love to rekindle your will to live, even in seemingly dire circumstances.

Please remember that healing happens every day. People recover from all kinds of stage IV cancers every day. Hope is here. Hope is now. Allow hope to energize your healing.

o o o

I have a final "white-coat-pilled" scene that I want to leave you with.

January 20, 2020, marks our first visit with an actual oncologist. As you know, on that day, we were told that Paul had stage IV lung cancer, that surgery was not possible, that Paul likely had four to six months to live without effective treatment, and that a best-case scenario was around two years.

Paul's oncologist was compassionate and empathetic. He had sympathy in his eyes and let us absorb the blow. Then, he said quietly, "I'm sorry."

After some further discussion, we left his office and went home. My heart and stomach sank to my feet as I cried convulsively: Paul was standing before me in our family room of the same in which I presently write.

"Four to six months," I sobbed.

"Becky," said Paul, calmly, steadily, yet forcefully. As we stood facing each other, he very purposefully held my arms down to my sides and said, "Look at me."

I looked into his tear-free, peaceful eyes. "What you just heard was a hex. Don't let it be a hex. We must reject it. It is not true. Otherwise, if we claim it and believe it, the effects will be like the witch doctor's voodoo."

As soon as those words—those words of *deep truth*—came from his mouth, commanding my hysteric convulsions to *be still*, I was still. I believed Paul. I knew it to be true. I calmed down. With this deep truth, I could be his partner and caregiver on the road before us, I could reject the words "four to six months," and I could reject the words "two years." I knew it did not have to be this way.

This is how Paul set me straight so that later, in his throes of chemotherapy, I could set *him* straight to turn things around and summon from him his will to live.

Paul is not a number. Paul is not a statistic. You are not a number. You are not a statistic. Paul is Paul, my husband, father of my child, a being uniquely wrought and wonderfully made—as are you, dear reader.

Paul wrote the book that we wished we had during that winter of 2020.

What he wrote here is true. I witnessed it.

May this book be a gift of life to the world and a gift of life and hope to *you* so that you too might have hope every day in every way.

With a vast and incomprehensible love for life,

Rebecca Kabler Boggs Seyferth, PhD

Acknowledgments

THE MOST IMPORTANT ACKNOWLEDGMENTS I CAN MAKE ARE TO MY wife, Rebecca, and my daughter, Jacqulyn. They know what they have been through for the past five years, and if you or a loved one has experienced cancer and cancer treatments, you have some idea of what they have gone through as well. You have met them in various passages of this book, but if you met either of them in person, you would understand why the exercise of my will to live, even during the worst of it, was not all that hard. All I had to do was think of them.

Many others made this book possible, some by treating me so that I might live long enough to write it. These individuals include, *inter alia*, the doctors and staff at Kansas University Cancer Center, MD Anderson Cancer Center, and Sperling Medical Center. I am especially grateful to three additional medical experts who treated me during the past five years: my lifelong friend Dr. Kenneth Haugen who kindly wrote the foreword to this book, and my new-found and now lifelong friends, integrative oncologist Dr. Lucas Tims and Chinese medicine expert Chris Powell.

In addition to these experts, I was blessed to have a draft or portions of a draft of this book reviewed by established authors whom I greatly respect and greatly benefitted from: Laurence Gonzales, David Von Drehle, and Jack Hitt. Along with these authors, many great friends and close family reviewed a draft of the book and offered helpful edits and suggestions: Mike Blumenthal, Bruce Moothart, Mark Haddad, Deena Jenab, Gene Graham, Chip Robertson, Jr., Marc and Laura Boggs, Robbie Boggs, Chip Boggs,

Sue Adams, Marianne Sun, Steve and Courtney Anderson, Tom and Jackie Shaver, Reverand Eric Williams, Rabbi Zalman Techtel, Nadine Beech, Jennifer Olson, Amanda Nerstaad, Jeff Chaney, and my three wonderful sisters—Kris Anderson, Sue Scraver, and Laurie Kroesing. Many thanks as well to Don Ipock, who used his professional talents on the photo on the back of the book. Other friends and family have listened patiently to mini-sermons on the topic of this book, and there are far too many of them to list here. Their patience and their feedback were most appreciated.

I also wish to thank my longtime colleagues Trynnel Ragsdale and Melissa Miller. Trynnel typed most of this manuscript and treated it like a brief to the Supreme Court, all while enduring many personal and family challenges. Melissa helped me track down other cancer survivors with her characteristic diligence and charmed some of them into being willing to talk to me. Trynnel and Melissa, like everybody else at the law firm of Seyferth, Blumenthal & Harris, LLC, are serious professionals who know how to get things done the right way.

Finally, I wish to mention once again my dear and now departed friend and mentor, Mark G. Flaherty. Mark and I discussed navigation of the deep waters of cancer survival at length, and many other worthy topics as well. He was a brilliant man, but his health situation was also "very grave" during the time this book was being written. Mark died on April 27, 2022. Mark's last words to me were simply "thank you." This is my belated thank-you to him. I can only hope that Mark would be pleased with at least some of the pages in this book.

Appendix:

The Twenty-One "Rules" of Deep Cancer Survival

If you are reading this book as one of the recently diagnosed, it is understandable that you may be looking for a simple guide for what to do *right now*.

What follows below is a nutshell of the "rules" of survival discussed in this book. Please note: these rules are really a series of suggested *actions:* each of them is entirely within your control, most of them do not cost anything, and many of them do not require a significant time commitment. The rules follow the chronological sequence used in this book, but the recently diagnosed cancer patient need not perform or ponder them in any sequential order.

Here are the rules:

Rule 1: Make the Decision to Fight
Rule 2: Become a Happy, Optimistic Warrior
Rule 3: Get a Second Opinion
Rule 4: Consciously Confront the "Meaning" of Your Diagnosis
Rule 5: Consciously Confront the Possibility of Death
Rule 6: Employ Visualization in Aid of Your Healing

o   o   o

Rule 7: Learn to Assess Survival Rates for Your Disease

Rule 8: Become a Self-Doctor and Citizen-Scientist

Rule 9: Learn How to Communicate with Doctors

Rule 10: Weigh the Possibilities of Complementary Medicine

Rule 11: Navigate the Mental Game of Scans

Rule 12: Weigh the Potential of Diets, Fasting, and Supplements

o o o

Rule 13: Set Realistic Goals for Your Treatments

Rule 14: Navigate the Paradox of Double Mind

Rule 15: Take Advantage of Remission

Rule 16: Deal with Recurrences and Second Cancers

Rule 17: Pass It On—Help Others with Cancer

Rule 18: Adjust Your Visualizations

o o o

Rule 19: Reject All Notions of "False Hope"

Rule 20: Create a "Special Deck" of Survivors with Your Disease

o o o

Rule 21: Incorporate Daily Autosuggestion into Your Healing

Each of these "rules" is examined and discussed in a separate chapter.

Each rule is worthy of your consideration, and *none* of these actions should, properly understood, lessen or contradict the effectiveness of your standard cancer treatments or replace them.

Bibliography

Al Achkar, Morhaf. *Roads to Meaning and Resilience with Cancer: Forty Stories of Coping, Finding Meaning and Building Resilience While Living with Incurable Lung Cancer*. Morhaf Al Achkar, 2019.

Apple, Sam. *Ravenous: Otto Warburg, the Nazis, and the Search for the Cancer-Diet Connection*. New York, Liveright Publishing Corporation, 2021.

Armstrong, C. Michael, and Eric A Vohr. *Cancer with Hope: Facing Illness, Embracing Life, and Finding Purpose*. Baltimore, MD: Johns Hopkins University Press, 2021.

Aurelius, Marcus. *Meditations*. S.L., Collectors Library, 2020.

Bashforth, Emily. "What Does Rebellious Hope Mean? How to Buy Dame Deborah James' T-Shirt." Metro, June 29, 2022. metro.co.uk/2022/06/29/what-does-rebellious-hope-mean-how-to-buy-dame-deborah-james-t-shirt-16913260/amp/.

Bauml, Joshua M., Andrea Troxel, C. Neill Epperson et al. "Scan-Associated Distress in Lung Cancer: Quantifying the Impact of "Scanxiety."" *Lung Cancer*, vol. 100, Oct. 2016, pp. 110–113, https://doi.org/10.1016/j.lungcan.2016.08.002. Accessed 7 Feb. 2021.

Bloch, Annette and Richard. *Fighting Cancer*. Kansas City, MO: RA Bloch Cancer Foundation, 2010.

Brooks, Cyrus Harry. *The Practice of Autosuggestion by the Method of Émile Coué*. New York City: Dodd, Mead & Company, 1922.

Christofferson, Travis. *Tripping over the Truth: The Return of the Metabolic Theory of Cancer Illuminates a New and Hopeful Path to a Cure*. Createspace, 2014.

Compass Oncology. "Cancer Survivors Helping Cancer Patients |
Compass Oncology." Accessed 19 Mar. 2024. www.compasson-
cology.com/cancer-survivorship/helping-others.

Douthat, Ross. *The Deep Places*. Convergent Books, 26 Oct. 2021.

Faria, Miguel, Monica Teixeira, Maria Joao Pinto, and Paulo Sargento.
"Efficacy of Acupuncture on Cancer Pain: A Systematic Review
and Meta-analysis." *Journal of Integrative Medicine* 22:3 (May
2024): 235–44.

Flanagan, Caitlin. "I Thought Stage IV Cancer Was Bad Enough."
The Atlantic, May 5, 2020. www.theatlantic.com/magazine/
archive/2020/06/surviving-cancer-coronavirus-pandemic/610594/.

———. "I'll Tell You the Secret of Cancer." *The Atlantic*, August
23, 2021. www.theatlantic.com/magazine/archive/2021/08/
caitlin-flanagan-secret-of-surviving-cancer/619844/.

Flick, Jim, and Jack Nicklaus. "Flick and Nicklaus: Go to the
Movies." *Golf Digest*, April 27, 2010, www.golfdigest.com/story/
flick-nicklaus-film.

Fung, Dr. Jason. *The Cancer Code*. HarperCollins, 10 Nov. 2020.

Gallwey, W. Timothy. *The Inner Game of Tennis*. New York City:
Random House, 2010.

García, Héctor, and Francesc Miralles. *The Book of Ichigo Ichie: The Art
of Making the Most of Every Moment, the Japanese Way*. New York
City: Penguin Books, 2019.

García, Héctor, and Francesc Miralles. "What Is
Ichigo Ichie? 10 Rules Of The Japanese Way To
Happiness." December 30, 2019. MindBodyGreen.
com. https://www.mindbodygreen.com/articles/
what-is-ichigo-ichie-10-rules-of-the-japanese-way-to-happiness.

Ge, Long, Qi Wang, Yihan He et al. "Acupuncture for Cancer Pain:
An Evidence-Based Clinical Practice Guideline." *Chinese
Medicine*, vol. 17, no. 1, 5 Jan. 2022. https://doi.org/10.1186/
s13020-021-00558-4.

Gonzales, Laurence. *Deep Survival: Who Lives, Who Dies, and Why: True Stories of Miraculous Endurance and Sudden Death*. New York City: W. W. Norton & Co, 2004.

Gould, Stephen Jay. "The Median Isn't the Message." *Journal of Ethics*, vol. 15, no. 1, Jan. 2013, 77–81. www.journalofethics.ama-assn. org/article/median-isn't-message/2013-01.

Greger, Michael. *How Not to Die*. New York City: Flatiron Books, 2015.

Guclu, Yusuf Adnan. "A Hope-Enhancement Instrument for Palliative Care Cancer Patients." *Cureus*, vol. 11, no. (8), 7 Aug. 2019, https://doi.org/10.7759/cureus.5342.

Guo, Huiru, Hegen Li, Lihua Zhu, Jiali Feng, Xiange Huang, and Jan P. A. Baak. "'How Long Have I Got?' in Stage IV NSCLC Patients with at Least 3 Months up to 10 Years Survival, Accuracy of Long-, Intermediate-, and Short-Term Survival Prediction Is Not Good Enough to Answer This Question." *Frontiers in Oncology*, vol. 11, 21 Dec. 2021. https://doi.org/10.3389/fonc.2021.761042.

Hillen, M. A., H. C. J. M. de Haes, L. J. A. Stalpers et al. "How Can Communication by Oncologists Enhance Patients Trust?" *Annals of Oncology*, Vol 25, Issue 4 (April 2014). https:www.annalsofon-cology.org/article/S0923-7534(19)36509-3/fulltext.

Hitchens, Christopher. *Mortality*. Twelve, 4 Sept. 2012.

Hjorleifsdottir, E. and D. E. Carter. "Communicating with Terminally Ill Cancer Patients and Their Families." *Nurse Education Today* 20 (2000), 646–653.

Hutschnecker, Arnold A. *The Will to Live*. New York City: Simon & Schuster, 1983.

Jacobs, Donald. *Patient Communication for First Responders and EMS Personnel*. Hoboken, NJ: Prentice Hall, 1991.

Johns Hopkins Medicine. "Imagery." Accessed July 15, 2024. www. hopkinsmedicine.org/health/wellness-and-prevention/imagery.

Kyriacou, D. N. "Evidence-Based Medical Decision Making: Deductive versus Inductive Logical Thinking." *Academic Emergency Medicine*, vol. 11, no. 6, 1 June 2004, 670–671. https://doi.org/10.1197/j.aem.2004.02.512.

Lloyd, Michael, *Beating Crazy Odds*. CreateSpace, 2014.

Longo, Valter, Maria Di Tano, Mark P. Mattson, and Novella Guidi. "Intermittent Fasting and Periodic Fasting, Longevity and Disease." *Natural Aging* 1 (2021): 47–59.

Love, Shayla. "The Power of the Nocebo Effect." Vice, March 27, 2019, www.vice.com/en/article/59xe9b/the-power-of-the-nocebo-effect-v26m1.

Lung Cancer Foundation of America. "Seeing Lung Cancer as a Chronic Disease: Michael Weitz's Story." Accessed March 18, 2024. lcfamerica.org/story/seeing-lung-cancer-as-a-chronic-disease/.

Lung Cancer Group. "Can Lung Cancer Go into Remission? Lung Cancer Remission Rates." Accessed March 18, 2024. www.lungcancergroup.com/lung-cancer/prognosis/remission.

Mao, Jun J., Christina Shearer Palmer, Kaitlin Elizabeth Healy et al. "Complementary and Alternative Medicine Use among Cancer Survivors: A Population-Based Study." *Journal of Cancer Survivorship : Research and Practice*, vol. 5, no. 1, March 1, 2011, 8–17, www.ncbi.nlm.nih.gov/pmc/articles/PMC3564962/, https://doi.org/10.1007/s11764-010-0153-7.

Mitchell, Felicia. "Remembering Cancer Role Models." Cure Today, August 15, 2018. www.curetoday.com/view/remembering-cancer-role-models.

Richard & Annette Bloch Family Foundation. "Multidisciplinary Second Opinion Centers." Accessed March 18, 2024. blochcancer.org/resources/multidisciplinary-second-opinion-centers/.

Mulhany, Nick. "1 in 12 Chance of Second Cancer in Many Survivors." *Medscape*. Accessed March 19, 2024. www.medscape.com/viewarticle/866433.

Musschenga, Bert. "Is There a Problem with False Hope?" *The Journal of Medicine and Philosophy: A Forum for Bioethics and Philosophy of Medicine*, vol. 44, no. 4, 29 July 2019, pp. 423–441, https://doi.org/10.1093/jmp/jhz010.

Nasha Winters, and Jess Higgins Kelley. *The Metabolic Approach to Cancer : Integrating Deep Nutrition, the Ketogenic Diet, and Nontoxic Bio-Individualized Therapies*. White River Junction, VT: Chelsea Green Publishing, 2017.

Roberts, Bernadette. *The Path to No-Self : Life at the Center*. Albany, N.Y., State University of New York Press,.

Rosenbaum, Ernest, and David Spiegel. "Hope as a Strategy." Surviving Cancer. Accessed March 18, 2024. med.stanford.edu/survivingcancer/cancers-existential-questions/hope-as-a-strategy.html.

Rosenbaum, Ernest H, and Isadora R Rosenbaum. *Cancer Supportive Care: The Complete Guide for Patients and Their Families*. South Brisbane, QLD: Somerville House Books, 1998.

———. *Inner Fire: Your Will to Live: Stories of Courage, Hope, and Determination*. Medford, NJ: Plexus Publishing, 1999.

Sabbage, Sophie. *The Cancer Whisperer: Finding Courage, Direction, and the Unlikely Gifts of Cancer*. New York City: Plume, An Imprint Of Penguin Random House, 2017.

Sabin, Glenn, and Dawn Lemanne. *n of 1*. Fon Press, 2016.

Sawada, Namie Okino, Márcia Maria Fontão Zago, Cristina Maria Galvão et al. "The Outcomes of Visualization and Acupuncture on the Quality of Life of Adult Cancer Patients Receiving Chemotherapy." *Cancer Nursing*, Vol. 33, No. 5, Sept. 2010, E21–E28. https://doi.org/10.1097/ncc.0b013e3181d86739

Schaefer, Brian. *Salvestrols: Journeys to Wellness*. CreateSpace, 2013.

Seiler, Annina, and Josef Jenewein. "Resilience in Cancer Patients." *Frontiers in Psychiatry*, Vol. 10, No. 208, April 5, 2019. https://doi.org/10.3389/fpsyt.2019.00208.

Seneca. *Seneca's Letters from a Stoic*. David & Charles, 2016.

Spiegel, David. "Mind Matters in Cancer Survival." *Psychooncology*, Vol. 21, No. 6, March 21, 2012. https://doi.org/10.1002/pon.3067.

Stroud, Les. *Will to Live*. New York City: HarperCollins, 2011.

Turner, Kelly A. *Radical Remission: Surviving Cancer against All Odds*. New York City: HarperOne, 2015.

American Cancer Society. "Understanding Statistics Used to Guide Prognosis and Evaluate Treatment." Cancer.net, April 8, 2010. www.cancer.net/navigating-cancer-care/cancer-basics/understanding-statistics-used-guide-prognosis-and-evaluate-treatment.

Varga, Katalin. *Beyond the Words: Communication and Suggestion in Medical Practice*. New York City: Nova Science Publishers, 2011.

W., Bill, et al. *Alcoholics Anonymous: The Big Book: The Original 1939 Edition*. Mineola, New York: Ixia Press, An Imprint Of Dover Publications, Inc, 2019.

W., Nila. "Stories, Coping with Metastatic Lung Cancer." CancerCare. Accessed March 19, 2024. www.cancercare.org/stories/22-nila_w.

Warren, Mark, and Tim Junod. "Why There Is Nothing False about 'False Hope.'" *Esquire*, January 21, 2014. www.esquire.com/news-politics/news/a32792/false-hope/.

Wilber, Ken. *A Theory of Everything*. Boulder, CO: Shambhala Publications, 2000.

———. *Grace and Grit*. Boulder, CO: Shambhala Publications, 2001.

Zasowska-Nowak, Anna, Piotr Jan, and Aleksandra Cialkowska-Rysz. "High-Dose Vitamin C in Advanced-Stage Cancer Patients." *Nutrients*, Vol. 13, No. 3 (February 26, 2021), 735. https://doi.org/10.3390/nu13030735.

Endnotes

Preface

1   Huiru Guo et al. "'How Long Have I Got?' in Stage IV NSCLC Patients with at Least 3 Months up to 10 Years Survival, Accuracy of Long-, Intermediate-, and Short-Term Survival Prediction Is Not Good Enough to Answer This Question," *Frontiers in Oncology*, 11, December 21, 2021, https://doi.org/10.3389/fonc.2021.761042.

2   Ernest H. Rosenbaum, MD, and Isadora R. Rosenbaum, MA, *Inner Fire: Your Will to Live* (Cancer Supportive & Survivorship Care, 2009), 9.

3   Laurence Gonzales, *Deep Survival: Who Lives, Who Dies, and Why: True Stories of Miraculous Endurance and Sudden Death* (New York City: W. W. Norton & Company, 2004), 170, quoting survival expert Kenneth Hill.

4   Ernest Rosenbaum, MD, and David Spiegel, MD, "Hope as a Strategy," accessed August 12, 2024, www.med.stanford.edu.

5   Annette and Richard Bloch, *Fighting Cancer* (Kansas City, MO: R.A. Bloch Cancer Foundation, 2010).

Background

6   Sidhartha Mukherjee, *Cancer: The Emperor of All Maladies* (New York: Scribner, 2010). Note, xviii: "In the end, cancer truly emerges , as a nineteenth-century surgeon once wrote in a book's frontispiece, as 'the emperor of all maladies, the king of terrors."

7   Gonzales, *Deep Survival*, 27.

8   Kelly Turner, *Radical Remission*, 285.

Treatment Background and Medical History

9   Kelly A. Turner, *Radical Remission: Surviving Cancer against All Odds* (New York City: HarperOne, 2015), 285.

10   Turner, *Radical Remission*, 6.

11   "Study of 'exceptional responders' Yields Clues to Cancer and Potential Treatments," www.cancer.gov, November 19, 2020, defining "exceptional responders " as "someone who had a partial or complete response to a treatment that would be effective in less than 10% of similar patients." Accessed by author August 12, 2024.

12   Glenn Sabin and Dawn Lemanne, MD, MPH, *n of 1* (Silver Spring, MD: Fon Press, 2016).

The Structure of This Book

13   Guo, "'How Long Have I Got?'" Throughout this chapter and the remainder of the book, I will be making repeated references to this article. The descriptions and quotations made throughout the remainder of the book are taken from pages 1–4 of the article. The interested reader would be well served by closely absorbing the specific data and conclusions within this article.

14   Guo, "'How Long Have I Got?'"

15   Guo, "'How Long Have I Got?'"

Part I. Rebellious Hope and the First Ninety Days

16   Gonzales, *Deep Survival*, 85.

17   Gonzales, *Deep Survival*, 218.

18   Rosenbaum, *Inner Fire*, 175.

19   Bloch, *Fighting Cancer*, 134.

20   Bloch, *Fighting Cancer*, 134.

21   Bloch, *Fighting Cancer*, 134–135.

22   Travis Christofferson, *Tripping over the Truth: How the Metabolic Theory of Cancer Is Overturning One of Medicine's Most Entrenched Paradigms* (Chelsea, VT: Chelsea Green Publishing, 2017), xv. This quote is from the foreword to the book by Dominic P. D'Agostino, PhD.

23   Peter Attia, *Outlive: The Science and Art of Longevity* (New York City: Harmony Publishing, 2023), 145.

24   Ernest H. Rosenbaum and Isadora R. Rosenbaum, *Inner Fire: Your Will to Live: Stories of Courage, Hope, and Determination* (Cancer Supportive & Survivorship Care, 2009).

25   Rosenbaums, *Inner Fire*, 84.

26   Rosenbaums, *Inner Fire*, 86.

27   Michael Lloyd, *Beating Crazy Odds* (CreateSpace, 2014), 1.

28   Turner, *Radical Remission*, 77.

29   Gonzales, *Deep Survival*, 219.

30   Lloyd, *Beating Crazy Odds*, 3.

31   Sophie Sabbage, *The Cancer Whisperer: Finding Courage, Direction, and the Unlikely Gifts of Cancer* (New York City: Plume/RandomHouse, 2017), 17–18.

32   Gonzales, *Deep Survival, 85.*

33   Bloch, *Fighting Cancer*, 17.

34   Gonzales, *Deep Survival*, 216.

35   Gonzales, *Deep Survival*, 177.

36   Stephen Jay Gould, "The Median Isn't the Message," *AMA Journal of Ethics*, accessed March 18, 2024, https://journalofethics.ama-assn.org/article/median-isnt-message/2013-01.

37   Gould, "The Median Isn't the Message."

38   Gould, "The Median Isn't the Message."

39   Richard and Annette Bloch Family Foundation, "Multidisciplinary Second Opinion Centers," updated April 11, 2013, accessed August 12, 2024, www.blochcancer.org.

40   Ken Wilber, *A Theory of Everything: An Integral Vision for Business, Politics, Science, and Spirituality by Ken Wilber* (Boulder, CO: Shambhala Publications, 2000).

41   Ken Wilber, *Grace and Grit: Spirituality and Healing in the Life of Treya Killam Wilber* (Dublin: Gill & Macmillan Ltd, 1994).

42   Wilber, *Grace and Grit*, 40.

43   Wilber, *Grace and Grit*, 40.

44   Wilber, *Grace and Grit*, 40.

45   Wilber, *Grace and Grit*, 41.

46   Wilber, *Grace and Grit*, 41.

47   Morhaf Al Achkar, MD, PhD, *Roads to Meaning and Resilience with Cancer: Forty Stories of Coping, Finding Meaning and Building Resilience While Living with Incurable Lung Cancer* (Morhaf Al Achkar, 2019), 2.

48   David Spiegel, "Mind Matters in Cancer Survival," *Psychooncology* 21(6)(June 2012): 588–593.

49   Turner, *Radical Remission*, 145.

50   Marcus Aurelius, *Meditations* (s.l. Collectors Library, 2020).

51   Gonzales, *Deep Survival*, 286, quoting Irwin Edman from the foreword to *Meditations* by Marcus Aurlieus, trans. George Long and ed. Irwin Edman (New York: Walter J. Black, 1945).

52   Turner, *Radical Remission*, 277.

53   Jim Flick and Jack Nicklaus, "Flick and Nicklaus: Go to the Movies," *Golf Digest*, April 27, 2010, accessed March 18, 2024, www.golfdigest.com/story/flick-nicklaus-film.

54   Namie Okino Sawada, Márcia Maria Fontão Zago, Cristina Maria Galvão et al., "The Outcomes of Visualization and Acupuncture on the Quality of Life of Adult Cancer Patients Receiving Chemotherapy," *Cancer Nursing*, vol. 33, no. 5 (Sept. 2010): E21–E28, https://doi.org/10.1097/ncc.0b013e3181d86739.

55   Liz Rolfe, Katja Schmidt, Edzard Ernst, "A Systematic
     Review of Guided Imagery as an Adjuvant Cancer Therapy,"
     Pyschooncology 14(8)(August 2005): 607–618.

56   Lloyd, *Beating Crazy Odds*, 56.

Part II. Responsible Hope: Surviving the First Year after Diagnosis

57   Yusuf Adnan Guclu, "A Hope-Enhancement Instrument for
     Palliative Care Cancer Patients," *Cureus*, vol. 11, no. 8, August 7,
     2019, https://doi.org/10.7759/cureus.5342.

58   Bloch, *Fighting Cancer*, x.

59   Guo, "'How Long Have I Got?'"

60   Shayla Love, "The Power of the Nocebo Effect," Vice,
     March 27, 2019, www.vice.com/en/article/59xe9b/
     the-power-of-the-nocebo-effect-v26m1.

61   Gould, "The Mean Isn't the Message," x.

62   Gould, "The Mean Isn't the Message."

63   Gould, "The Mean Isn't the Message."

64   Turner, *Radical Remission*, 37.

65   Ross Douthat, *The Deep Places: A Memoir of Illness and Discovery*
     (New York City: Convergent/RandomHouse, 2021).

66   Douthat, *The Deep Places*, 108.

67   Douthat, 108.

68   Glenn Sabin, *n of 1*, 113.

69   E. Hjorleifsdottir and D. E. Carter, "Communicating with
     Terminally Ill Cancer Patients and Their Families," *Nurse
     Education Today* 20 (2000), 646–653.

70   Dr. Jason Fung, *The Cancer Code* (New York City: HarperCollins,
     2020), 125.

71   Fung, *The Cancer Code*, 127.

72   D. N. Kyriacou, "Evidence-Based Medical Decision Making: Deductive versus Inductive Logical Thinking," *ACAD Emergency Med*. Vol. 11, No. 6. (June 2004), 670, https://doi.org/10.1197/j. aem.2004.02.512.

73   Jun James Mao, Christina Shearer Palmer, Kaitlin Elizabeth Healy et al., "Complementary and Alternative Medicine Use Among Cancer Survivors: A Population Based Study, *Journal of Cancer Survivorship*, March 20115(1):8–17.

74   Long Ge, Qi Wang, Yihan He et al., "Acupuncture for Cancer Pain: An Evidence-Based Clinical Practice Guideline," *Chinese Medicine* 17 (2022): 8.

75   Miguel Faria, Monica Teixeira, Maria Joao Pinto, and Paulo Sargento, "Efficacy of Acupuncture on Cancer Pain: A Systematic Review and Meta-analysis," *Journal of Integrative Medicine* 22:3 (May 2024): 235–244.

76   Anna Zasowska-Nowak, Piotr Jan Nowak, and Aleksandra Cialkowska-Rysz, "High-Dose Vitamin C in Advanced-Stage Cancer Patients," *Nutrients* 13(3)(March 2021): 735.

77   Gonzales, *Deep Survival*, 239.

78   Seneca, *Seneca's Letters from a Stoic* (David & Charles, 2016).

79   Turner, *Radical Remission*, 15.

80   Sam Apple, *Ravenous: Otto Warburg, the Nazis, and the Search for the Cancer-Diet Connection* (New York City: Liveright Publishing Corporation, 2021), 318.

81   Apple, *Ravenous*, 318.

82   Apple, *Ravenous*, 318.

83   Nasha Winters and Jess Higgins Kelley, *The Metabolic Approach to Cancer: Integrating Deep Nutrition, the Ketogenic Diet, and Nontoxic Bio-Individualized Therapies* (White River Junction, VT: Chelsea Green Publishing, 2017).

84   Fung, *The Cancer Code*, 286.

85   Valter Longo, Maria Di Tano, Mark P. Mattson, and Novella
      Guidi, "Intermittent Fasting and Periodic Fasting, Longevity
      and Disease," *Natural Aging* 1 (2021): 47–59.

86   See Part F, the ECM

87   Fung, *The Cancer Code*, 197–201.

88   Turner, *Radical Remission*, 105.

89   Michael Greger, MD, *How Not to Die: Discover the Foods
      Scientifically Proven to Prevent and Reverse Disease* (New York
      City: Flatiron Books, 2015), 39.

90   Brian Schaefer, *Salvestrols: Journeys to Wellness* (CreateSpace,
      2013), 69.

Part III. Resilient Hope— Surviving Years Two through Five

91   Guo, "'How Long Have I Got?'"

92   Fung, *The Cancer Code*, 239.

93   Fung, *The Cancer Code*, 239.

94   Fung, *The Cancer Code*, 239.

95   Caitlin Flanagan, "I'll Tell You the Secret of Cancer," *The Atlantic*,
      August 23, 2021, www.theatlantic.com/magazine/archive/2021/08/
      caitlin-flanagan-secret-of-surviving-cancer/619844/.

96   Gonzales, *Deep Survival*, 205.

97   Christopher Hitchens, *Mortality* (New York City: Twelve Books,
      2012), 14.

98   Hitchens, *Mortality*.

99   Gonzales, *Deep Survival*, 218, quoting survival expert John
      Leach.

100   Bernadette Roberts, *The Path to No-Self: Life at the Center* (New
      York City: State University of New York Press, 1991).

101   Sabbage, *The Cancer Whisperer*, 11.

102   "Lung Cancer Remission," www.lungcancergroup.com.

103   Gonzales, *Deep Survival*, 119.

104   Annina Seiler and Josef Jenewein, "Resilience in Cancer
      Patients," *Frontiers in Psychiatry*, vol. 10, no. 208 (April 5, 2019),
      https://doi.org/10.3389/fpsyt.2019.00208.

105   Meghan O'Rourke, *The Invisible Kingdom: Reimagining Chronic
      Illness* (New York City: Riverhead Books, 2022), 257.

106   Héctor García and Francesc Miralles, "What Is Ichigo Ichie?
      10 Rules Of The Japanese Way To Happiness," December
      30, 2019, https://www.mindbodygreen.com/articles/
      what-is-ichigo-ichie-10-rules-of-the-japanese-way-to-happiness.

107   Nick Mulhany, "1 in 12 Chance of Second Cancer in Many
      Survivors," Medscape, June 21, 2016, https://www.medscape.
      com/viewarticle/866433.

108   Lynn Eldridge, "What Is Lung Cancer Recurrence," VeryWell
      Health, June 2022.

109   Rosenbaums, *Inner Fire*, 174.

110   Rosenbaums, *Inner Fire*, 174.

111   Lung Cancer Foundation of America, "An Amazing NSCLC
      Advocate: Meet Colleen Conner Ziegler," accessed August 15,
      2024, www.lcfamerica.org.

112   Bill W., *Alcoholics Anonymous: The Big Book: The Original 1939
      Edition* (Mineola, New York: Ixia Press, An Imprint Of Dover
      Publications, Inc, 2019).

113   Bill W., *Alcoholics Anonymous: The Big Book*, 89.

114   Lloyd, *Beating Crazy Odds*, 56.

115   O'Rourke, *The Invisible Kingdom*, 160.

Part IV. Replenished Hope and Survivor Role Models

116   Mark Warren and Tom Junod, "Why There Is Nothing False
      about 'False Hope,'" *Esquire*, January 21, 2014, www.esquire.
      com/news-politics/newsa32792/false-hope.

117 Lindsay B. Yeates, PhD, "Émile Coué and His Method (I): The Chemist of Thought and Human Action," *Australian Journal of Clinical Hypnotherapy & Hypnosis*, Vol 38, No 1 (Autumn 2016), 3–27.

118 Guo, "'How Long Have I Got?'"

119 Guo, "'How Long Have I Got?'"

120 Julie Radico, "Roads to Meaning and Resilience with Cancer," *Family Medicine* 52, no. 5 (2020): 373–374.

121 www.morhafalalachkar.com.

122 Lloyd, *Beating Crazy Odds*, 1.

123 Lloyd, *Beating Crazy Odds*, 109.

124 www.beatingcrazyodds.com.

125 Bloch, *Fighting Cancer*, 32–33.

126 Rosenbaums, *Inner Fire*, 84.

127 Rosenbaums, *Inner Fire*, 86.

128 Rosenbaums, *Inner Fire*, 89.

129 Jennifer Olson, interview with author, May 2024.

130 Olson, interview.

131 Olson, interview.

132 Olson, interview.

133 Olson, interview.

134 Savio P. Clemente, "Amanda Nerstad: I Survived Cancer and Here Is How I Did It," Medium, October 15, 2021.

135 Clemente, "Amanda Nerstad: I Survived Cancer and Here Is How I Did It."

136 www.diagnostics.roche.com.

137 www.diagnostics.roche.com.

138 Amanda Nerstad, "Survivor: Anyone with Lungs Can Get Lung Cancer," February 5, 2019, www.mdanderson.org.

Part V. **Rekindling Hope—Every Day, In Every Way**

139 Yeates, "Émile Coué and His Method," x.

140 Timothy W. Gallwey, *The Inner Game of Tennis* (New York City: Random House, 2010), 5–6.

141 Katalin Varga, "Suggestive Techniques Connected to Medical Interventions," *Interventional Medicine & Applied Science* 5(3) (September 2013): 95–100.

142 Katalin Varga, "Suggestive Techniques Connected to Medical Interventions," *Interventional Medicine & Applied Science* 5(3) (September 2013): 95–100.

143 Varga, "Suggestive Techniques Connected to Medical Interventions," 95.

144 Varga, "Suggestive Techniques Connected to Medical Interventions," 95–96.

145 Varga, "Suggestive Techniques Connected to Medical Interventions," 96.

146 Cyrus Harry Brooks, *The Practice of Autosuggestion by the Method of Émile Coué* (Dodd, Mead & Company, 1922), 55–56.

Will To Live—Walls of Hope, Inc.

THE PROCEEDS OF ALL SALES OF THIS BOOK WILL BE FOR A 501(c)3 charitable organization called Will To Live—Walls of Hope, Inc. Rebecca and I formed this organization in the spring of 2024. The purpose of this organization is to fund a "Wall of Hope" in every oncology center in the Kansas City community and beyond Kansas City. These Walls of Hope are available for review and to inspire hope for those going through cancer treatments and consist of the survival stories of those treated in such cancer centers.

The first Wall of Hope was installed at the University of Kansas Cancer Center in Westwood, Kansas, in the fall of 2024.

www.ingramcontent.com/pod-product-compliance
Lightning Source LLC
Chambersburg PA
CBHW031502120626
46545CB00005B/1717